Stretching Smarter
Stretching Healthier

Jolie Bookspan, M.Ed, Ph.D., FAWM

Quick, effective techniques
to stop injuries and increase flexibility

ISBN: 0-9721214-6-3

Check with your doctor
and use your brain
before using anything presented here

Dedication

To my grandmother, who stretched upside down, standing on one arm. I thought everyone's grandmother did that.

To my mother, who taught me how important it is to stretch right (and what happens to bad children who stretch wrong). She stretched upside down on one arm, too. She wanted me to stretch so that I'd be tall.

To my saint of a husband Paul. It's been over 32 years together and you still are, and have always been, my hero. At over 6' 9" tall, the stretching must have worked.

Foreword

by Audrey Tannenbaum, M.Ed, ATC, C.S.C.S., Certified Athletic Trainer, Certified Strength and Conditioning Specialist, Maccabean Games Triathlon Gold Medalist Practitioner of the Academy of Functional Exercise Medicine (AFEM).

To achieve balance in life, we must be flexible mentally, emotionally, and physically. "Stretching Smarter Stretching Healthier" address a long misunderstood topic—proper stretch technique. Dr. Bookspan explains and illustrates in an easy understandable way, proper effective stretches that will eliminate unnecessary joint trauma, potential injuries, and the pain that results from improper stretching. This book is fun and easy to read, while providing vital information about the importance of proper stretching, and the positive effects flexibility can have on joint health and quality of life.

Dr. Bookspan's passion for proper body mechanics has helped countless individuals. Once introduced to Dr. Bookspan's methods by following her simple instructions and common sense approach, the results are almost instant—pain reduction and pain free movement. Dr. Bookspan has changed my life for the better. I not only practice her techniques for stretching (and strengthening) in my personal training routine, but use them routinely as a training and rehabilitation tool in my professional role as an athletic trainer.

I am honored to have been given the privilege, not only to write the foreword for this book, but also to have been afforded the opportunity to know and learn from Dr. Bookspan. I can attribute my pain free movement and increased physical performance to her philosophy on proper stretch, posture, and movement technique. In today's "information age" it is difficult to know what to believe and what truly works. If you are as skeptical as I, let me reassure you that the truth is in this book, "Stretching Smarter Stretching Healthier."

Table of Contents

Introduction

Many people don't gain flexibility even with constant stretching. Other people stretch to reduce pain or injuries but are injured during activity, on the job, or even from their stretching. The problem seems to be how people stretch then how they exercise and go about their "real life" outside of the gym and their stretching routine. This book will show you how to make a few simple changes to:

- Stop hurting yourself from bad stretching
- Change unhelpful, unhealthy stretches to healthy beneficial stretches
- Reduce stiffness, muscle strain, back pain, and other joint pain
- Retrain your body to move in healthy ways in real life
- Build good stretches into your daily life (functional stretching)
- Re-educate your muscles and joints to not get tight and strained in the first place.
- Stretch your brain so that you are not just doing a bunch of stretches, but understanding how your body and stretching work

Stiffness and pain are not normal consequences of aging. At the same time, being more flexible alone is not what improves your health or reduces pain. With the information in this book, you will learn how to stretch smarter and stretch healthier, and apply good stretches and healthy movement to all you do. Have fun choosing from the many fun stretches in this book.

Quadriceps Stretch, Standing

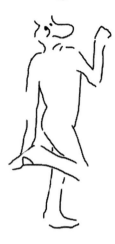

Problem:

- Check if you do this stretch with the leg bent at the front where it meets the body, or with increased inward curve in the lower back. These decrease stretch in the muscles of the front of the hip and thigh, and the purpose of the stretch—to lengthen the front hip muscles—is lost.

Quick Fix:

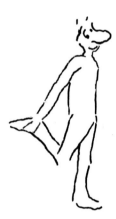

- Tuck your hip under, as if starting an "abdominal crunch." Don't curl your upper body forward; just tilt your hip under to reduce the lower back arch. The pelvis becomes vertical along the "side seam." Done right, you will immediately feel the stretch move to your thigh. Straighten your arm and push your knee downward and backward, easily, not so far that it hurts.

- The point of the stretch is to lengthen the front of your hip, not bend it. Instead of bending the leg forward to reach your foot, stand straight, lift your foot behind you, and reach back. If you are too tight to reach your foot, place it on a chair or bench behind you. Work up from there.

Quadriceps Stretch, Sitting and Lying Down

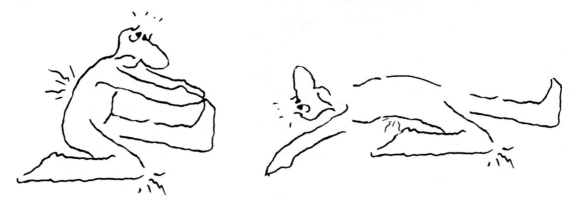

Problem:

- Check if you do this by stretch twisting the knee, instead of rotating the thigh from the hip. The knee joint is not shaped to twist much, but open and close like a hinge. Several problems can happen. Ligaments that hold the leg bones together like straps at each side of the knee can overstretch and no longer hold snugly, creating unstable, loose knee joint. Two small cushions called menisci between the upper and lower leg bones can grind as the knee twists. When lying back, the back of the thigh pressing on the calf muscle can pry the knee joint open a bit, particularly if you have thick legs.

Quick Fix:

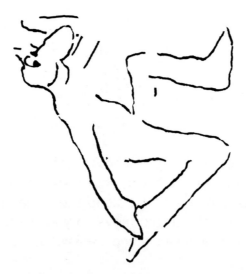

- Lie on your side. Bend both knees toward your chest, curling your body.

- Rest your head on your bottom arm, if you prefer.

- Keep your bottom leg bent in front of you. Bring your top leg behind you.

- Roll your shoulder back. Push your foot away from your body into your hand, instead of pulling your foot toward your body with your hand. Straighten your arm. Relax. Breathe. If you can't reach your foot with your hand, just rest with your leg bent behind you. Enjoy stretching.

- Drop your knee toward the floor and raise to vary the stretch.

- Keep breathing. Relax and let the muscles lengthen. Hold for a few seconds and change sides.

- Do this quadriceps stretch any time you are lying down, for example, to watch television, or before falling asleep in bed.

Brain Stretch:

- It's not true that pulling your foot away from your body makes you arch your back. You control whether your back arches by using your torso muscles. Tuck your hip under you to reduce the arch.

Why Stretch Your Front Leg and Hip Muscles?

- Many people keep their hip bent all day sitting, then continue when standing and for common exercises. They train and practice restricted, faulty movement, pelvis tilted forward, and short anterior hip muscles.

- Tight front hip and leg muscles contribute to bent standing position, adding to lower back pain and hip dysfunction.

Use The Quadriceps Stretch for Healthier Standing Posture in Daily Life:

- Stretch to retrain yourself to lengthen the front of the hip so you don't stand bent forward at the hip where your leg meets your body.

- By straightening, not keeping the front of your hip bent, you get a free, built-in stretch for your hip, and stop tightness that produces painful pinching from overarched lower back when trying to stand or lie flat.

Brain Stretch:

- If your front hip and thigh are so tight that you cannot stand up or lie flat without bent hip or lumbar arching, you will go about your daily activities in tight arched (hyperlordotic) posture, which is one of the major causes of lower back pain. Even with stretched muscles, you still need to hold neutral spine yourself so that you don't sag.

Achilles Tendon Stretch

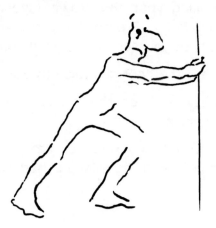

Problem:

- This "lunge and lean" stretch is commonly done with the back foot turned out, the body tilted forward, and the lower back arched. The stretch on the Achilles tendon and calf muscle in the back of the lower leg is diminished or lost.

Quick Fix:

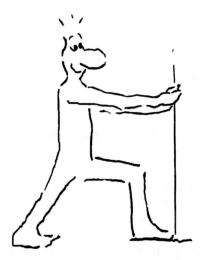

- Although the common "lunge and lean" is not the best way to stretch the Achilles tendon, to prevent it from being completely ineffective, hold your back foot straight. Don't let it turn out, not even a little. Look down to check your back foot. Straighten it. You will immediately feel a change in the stretch.

- Keep your heel down on the floor and straighten your back knee without locking it backward.

- Push your hip forward toward the wall, as if trying to touch your hip to the wall. Don't arch your back to lean the hip forward.

Quick Fix #2 for Achilles Tendon Stretch

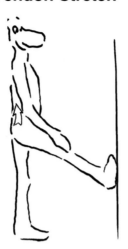

- The Achilles tendon wall stretch is a better stretch than the standard "lunge and lean." Stand facing the wall and press one heel against the wall at about knee height.

- Keep your standing foot forward, not turned out. Look down and check. Straighten it to face directly forward.

- Stand upright; don't lean or tilt forward. Don't let your hip curl under or your back round. Lift your chest and straighten your body.

Common Problems:

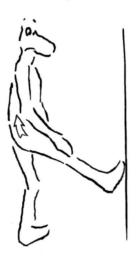

Several common habits make the stretch ineffective:
- Turning your standing foot out.
- Curling your hip under.
- Rounding your back.
- Not pressing your heel toward the wall.

Quick Fix #3 for Achilles Tendon Stretch

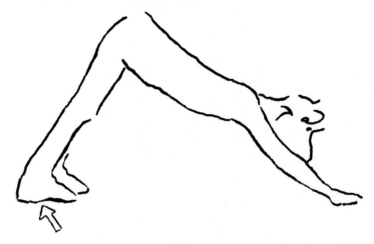

- "Downward dog," also called "downward facing dog," is a quick, effective stretch that stretches several areas including Achilles tendon. Start in a pushup position. Lift your hips upward and backward. Press your heels downward, knees straight, not locked.

- Keep your feet straight, not turned out; not even a little. Look down and see if your feet are parallel and facing straight forward. Keep weight on the outside rims of the feet, not sinking inward on the arches.

- Distribute weight on your whole hand. Avoid compressing your wrists.

- Don't let your hip curl under. Straighten your back and lift your chest.

Common Problems:

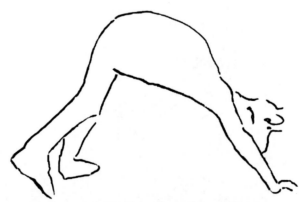

Several common habits make the stretch ineffective:

- Turning your feet out and letting weight fall inward on the arches.

- Curling your hip under so that your back rounds.

- Bending the knees too much

- Keeping weight back on the legs, not forward on the arms.

Quick Fix #4 for Achilles Tendon Stretch

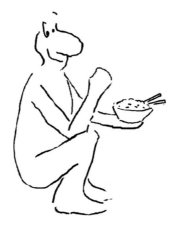

- Use the squat for a quick, effective Achilles tendon (and lower back) stretch when you sit to rest or stoop for chores. Keep your heels down, touching the floor.

- Keep your weight back toward your heels not leaning forward toward your toes.

- Keep weight distributed along the soles of your feet, not sinking inward on your arches.

- Keep your feet and knees facing the same direction, to avoid twisting the knee joint.

Common Problems:

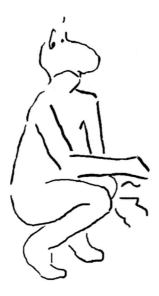

- Don't rock forward onto your toes, which shifts your weight through your knee joint and increases weight and force on your knee.

- Don't lift your heels, which reduces or eliminates the stretch.

Partner Achilles Tendon Stretch

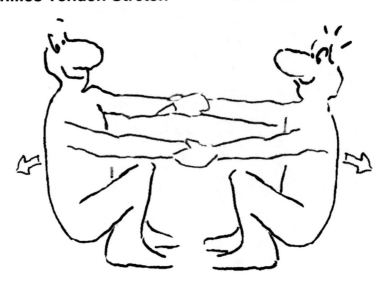

- Face a partner, arm's length away. Hold each other's hands, wrists, or forearms, whichever is comfortable. Bend knees while leaning back.

- Keep heels touching the floor as you lower. Don't lean forward onto the ball of your foot or lift your heels from the floor.

- Straighten your elbows and lean back onto your heels. Don't bend your elbows or pull your arms toward yourself. Just relax your weight back, holding each other's arms. You will feel a wonderful stretch in the back of your legs, in your hips, and your back.

Why Stretch Your Achilles?

- Tight Achilles tendon contributes to turning the foot outward. Turning outward unequally pressures your knee, ankle, and big toe when you walk. Walking with feet facing straight gives natural stretch to your Achilles tendon and reduces compression on your big toe, foot, ankle, and knee.

- If you turn your foot out, the push-off" of walking and running falls on the side of the big toe, instead of the ball of the foot. Turning out reduces "spring in the step," reduces jumping distance and running speed, and pushes your big toe toward the other toes with every step, increasing tendency to bunion.

- Tight Achilles tendon contributes to faulty walking and moving habits that can further tighten the Achilles and bottom of the foot, increasing tendency to Achilles tendon pulls, tears, and plantar fasciitis.

Get Natural Built-In Achilles Tendon Stretch During Daily Life:

- Walking and moving with your feet facing straight forward gives a built-in functional stretch with each step. Retrain yourself to keep feet comfortably straight when standing and walking.

- When you go up the stairs, keep your heel down on the upper stair as you step up, not just the ball of the foot. This uses leg muscles instead of shifting weight to the front of the knee, and gives a built-in Achilles tendon stretch with each step.

- Whenever you bend to reach or pick up any object, keep your heels on the floor and your body upright. Keep your weight back toward your heels. You will save your back and knees, strengthen your muscles, and get effective stretches for your foot, Achilles tendon, and calf muscles.

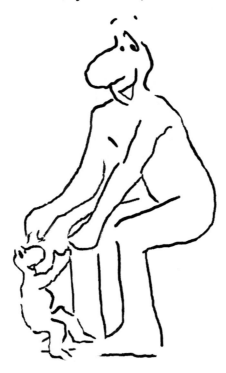

Brain Stretch:

- A few Achilles stretches won't "undo" a day of walking and bending in ways that tighten your legs and feet. Use good walking and bending for healthy, built-in Achilles tendon, leg, and foot stretching.

Inside Leg Stretch, Sitting

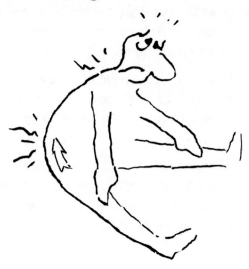

Problem:

- Check if you sit with your back rounded and pelvis/hip tipped backward. Sitting rounded does not stretch the hamstrings or inner leg muscles much, but puts high pressure on the discs of the lower back. It also practices poor rounded posture that you already may be overdoing at your computer, desk, and other activities of daily living.

Quick Fix:

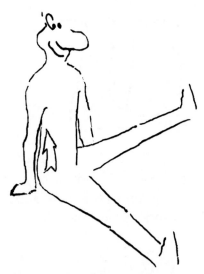

- Put your hands behind you. Push up to take your weight off your lower back. You will immediately feel the stretch shift to your legs.

- Sit upright and straight. Don't round your back, not even a little. Lift your chest. Pivot pelvis to upright, not tilted back. You will feel more stretch sitting upright and straight than rounding forward.

Quick Fix #2 for Inside Leg Stretch:

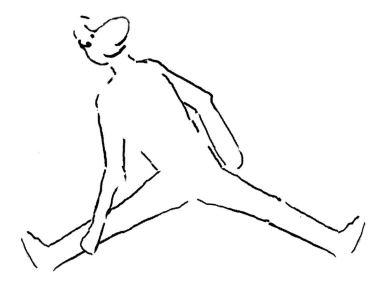

- When stretching to each side, don't face toward your leg. Sit upright and turn your back to the leg.

- Lean your back toward the leg, lifting your chest upward.

- You will feel more stretch sitting up straight and leaning back, than leaning forward rounded toward your leg.

Quick Fix #3 for Inside Leg Stretch

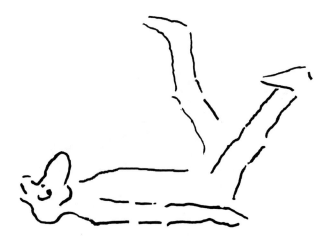

- Lie flat with legs overhead. Stretch your legs comfortably apart. Keep your head, shoulders, and backside lying flat, not lifting or rounding from the floor.

- This stretch can also be done by resting your legs against a wall while lying on the floor or bed. Don't lift the backside up. Stay flat.

Inside Leg Stretch, Standing

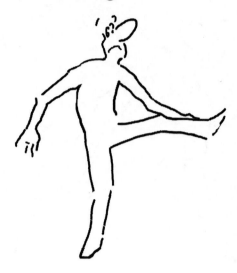

Problem:

- Check how you stand when lifting or kicking your leg. See if you let your back round and hip tilt under, if the standing leg pulls forward, or the knee sags inward. Poor position reduces stretch on the hamstrings and inner leg muscles. Spine rounding increases load on the lumbar discs, and pulling inward on the standing leg deforms the joint. You are practicing unhealthy rounded back posture that you already may be overdoing at your computer, desk, and during other daily activities.

Quick Fix:

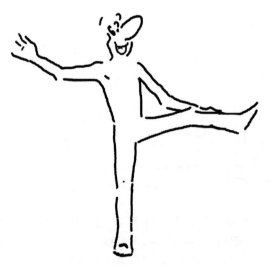

- Lower the lifted leg if you need, but stand upright and straight. Don't round your back, not even a little, to reach your leg. Lift your chest. You will get more stretch standing straight than bending over rounded.

- Relax your shoulders down and pull them back. Keep the foot of the standing leg facing straight forward. Don't let your hip curl under. Keep your knee of the standing leg straight, but not locked straight.

Brain Stretch:

- If you are so tight that your standing legs pulls forward at the hip, or inward at the knee when you raise the other leg, the front of your hip is too tight, putting you at risk for groin pulls and falling down when doing kicks or taking quick big steps. You are too tight to take a big step without your hip and lower back being yanked during daily activities.

- To stretch and lengthen your front hip muscles, use anterior hip stretches on pages 43-52.

Inside Leg Stretch, Balancing

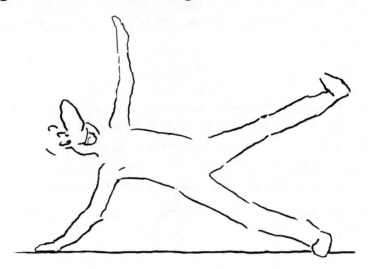

- From a pushup position, turn to the side to balance on one hand and one foot. Hold your body straight without sagging toward the floor. Breathe normally and raise your top leg as high as you can.

- Keep your weight distributed over your entire hand, not resting only on your wrist. Push your hand toward your fingertips to help lift you. Your arm does not need to be vertical, which puts your weight directly over your wrist.

- Don't lock your elbow straight, keep it slightly bent to keep your weight on your arm muscles, not your elbow joint.

- Keep your weight on the side and bottom of your standing foot, not just on the side of your ankle.

Brain Stretch:

- If your core muscles are so weak that you cannot hold your body straight without your torso sagging, it is likely that you will not be able to hold your body in healthy position just to get through your normal daily activities.

- Lying on the floor and bending forward to do "oblique crunches" does not train you how to hold your torso straight against sideways sagging and slouching. Instead, use this functional exercise to train your oblique and other torso muscles to keep you in healthy position against loads. Then transfer this knowledge to your daily life to stand straight when walking, standing, and carrying packages and loads on one hip.

Inside Leg Stretch, Knees Bent (Butterfly Stretch)

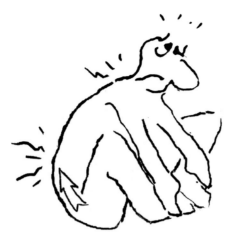

Problem:

- When you sit, notice if you sit with your rounded and the pelvis tipped backward. Stretching this way does not stretch your hip or inner leg muscles much, but puts high load on the discs of the lower back. It also practices poor rounded posture that you already may be overdoing at your computer, desk, and other activities of daily living.

Quick Fix:

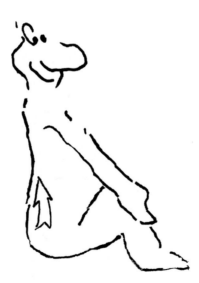

- Hold your shins and lift your upper body upward. Move your pelvis to vertical, not slouched back. Don't round your back, not even a little.

- You will feel more stretch sitting upright than leaning forward with rounded back and shoulders.

Brain Stretch—Use The Sitting Stretch for Healthier Spine Positioning in Daily Life:

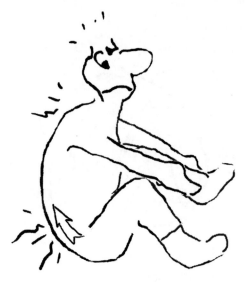

- When sitting to put on shoes and socks, sitting to do foot care (or sitting for anything else), don't let your hip curl under and your back round. Keep your back straight and chin in to get a free hip and inner leg stretch during everyday life activities like dressing.

- For putting on trousers, shoes and socks, standing gives effective hip and leg stretch while improving balance and daily function. Try the standing hip stretch on page 54.

Quick Fix #2 for Inside Leg Stretch—Using a Wall

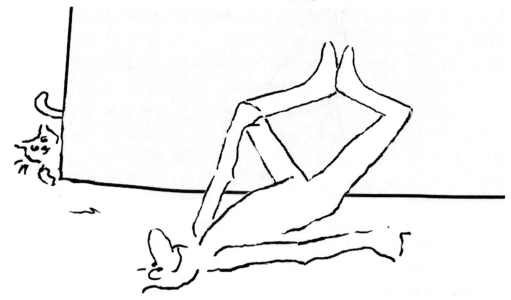

- Lie face up on the floor with the soles of your feet together, propped up on a wall, and your knees apart. Your backside touches the wall.

- Press your knees away with your hands to increase the stretch.

- Don't let your hips rise from the floor or round under you. Keep both hips flat on the floor.

- Lie flat without rounding your back or lifting your head or shoulders. By keeping your back, shoulders, and head on the floor, you train straight body position, and reduce load on the discs of your lower back.

Quick Fix #3 for Inside Leg Stretch—Rocket Ship Stretch

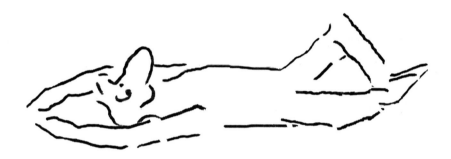

- Lie flat, face up, to get as good or better stretch for the inside of the leg as the sitting stretch, without the forward rounding and load on your lower back discs that occurs with bad sitting.

- Lie flat with your feet together and knees facing outward. Don't let your lower back increase in arch. To fix overarch, press lower spine toward the floor. Your knees may come upward. That's OK. That is learning how to get the stretch from the intended muscles, not from arching the lower back. Don't force at the hip.

- To increase the functional stretch for your whole body, put your arms by your ears, hands resting on the ground above your head.

- Don't arch your back to raise your arms. If your ribs or lower back lifts upward when you put arms overhead, your shoulders are tight—too tight to reach shelves and other overhead positions during daily life without overarching and pressuring your lower back. Use the pectoral stretch on pages 61-62 and shoulder stretches on pages 65-69 to increase resting length of the muscles. Then, remember not to lift the lower back upward instead of stretching from the shoulder and hip.

Quick Fix #4 for Inside Leg Stretch—Rocket Ship Legs Crossed

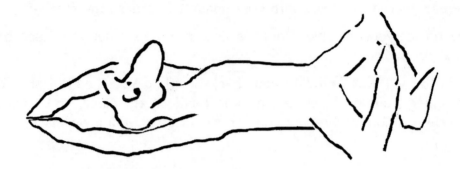

- Lie face up with knees bent and facing out. Cross your lower legs next to, but not on top of each other. Remove your shoes to allow room for your feet.

- To increase the functional stretch for your body, put your arms by your ears, hands resting on the ground.

- This rocket ship stretch with legs crossed is also a good "quick fix" for the cross-legged stretch, next.

Inside Leg Stretch, Cross-Legged

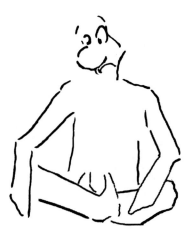

Problem:

- This stretch is commonly done with the ankles turned upward. By turning the ankles, you diminish the stretch on your hip and inner leg muscles, and put stretch force on the outside of your ankle. The outside of the ankle is not supposed to stretch much; it is supposed to hold your ankle straight so that it does not turn when you stumble. Overstretching the outside of your ankle can predispose you to ankle sprains.

Quick Fix:

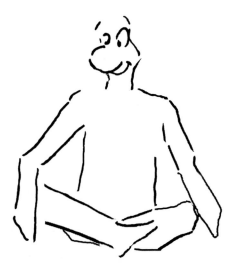

- Straighten your ankles to stop overstretching the outer ligaments. You will feel more stretch in your hip when you straighten your ankle.

- Sit upright. Don't round your back or let your hip tip back. Lift your chest. You will feel more stretch, and practice better habits by sitting up straight than by leaning forward with your back and shoulders rounded.

Hamstring Stretch, Standing

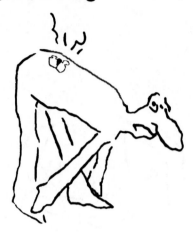

Problem:

- You already know that bending over forward to pick up a package puts herniating forces on the discs of your lower back. Bending over to stretch makes the same conditions. It is also not highly effective to stretch your hamstrings. Bending over to touch toes is a common, hidden contributor to back pain, whether you keep your back rounded or straight—the opposite of what people think they will achieve by hamstring stretching.

Why Common Hamstring Stretches Hurt the Vertebral Discs:

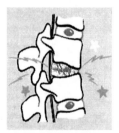

- Discs are tough cushions between your backbones. When you bend forward, the front of your vertebrae come closer together. The space between the back of your vertebrae opens. Like squeezing the front of a water balloon, the softer interior contents eventually move and bulge toward the back. Since discs are tough, it takes years of unequal squeezing for the contents to push outward to the back.

- After years of bad lifting, sitting slouched forward, and stretching by leaning over forward, the discs break down (degenerate) and move outward to the back (slip or herniate). Herniation can continue until it causes back pain, until the disc moves backward enough to touch nerves going down your leg causing sciatica and other nerve pain, or even press on your spinal cord. Discs are living body parts that can usually heal without surgery if you change to bend, and lift, and sit in healthy ways.

Quick Fix #1 for Standing Hamstring Stretch:

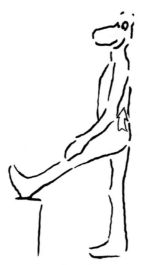

- Put the stretching leg directly in front of you, not out to the side. Keep the standing foot straight, not turned out. Look down to make sure your foot is completely straight.

- You will immediately feel the stretch move to your hamstring.

- Stand straight. Don't round your back, not even a bit. Lift your chest. You will feel more stretch standing straight than leaning forward with your back and shoulders rounded.

Common Problems:

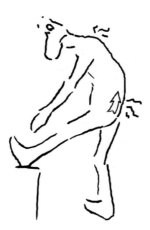

- Not facing straight toward your stretching leg.

- Turning your standing foot toe-out. Even a small turnout reduces or stops the stretch.

- Curling your hip under. Bending the standing leg by curling the hip under brings the hip forward, which reduces the stretch and increases pressure on the lower back. It also reinforces slouching and spine-rounding habits.

Quick Fix #2 for Standing Hamstring Stretch:

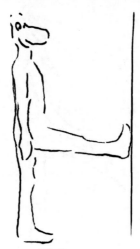

- Instead of bending over to stretch, or standing with one foot propped up, a more effective and functional hamstring stretch is to stand facing a wall and press one heel toward the wall at about hip height.

- Keep your standing foot straight, not turned out; not even a little. Glance down and see if your back foot is facing directly ahead.

- Lift your chest and stand straight. Don't let your hip curl under. Smile and breathe. Hold a few seconds and switch legs.

Common Problems:

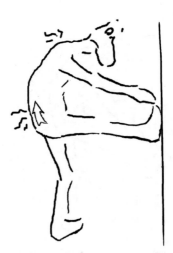

- Turning your standing foot out.
- Rounding your back.
- Curling your hip under. Bending the standing leg by curling the hip under brings the hip forward, which reduces the stretch, and reinforces slouching and spine-rounding habits.

Hamstring Stretch, Sitting

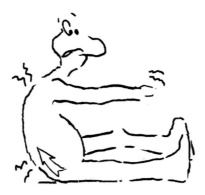

Problem:

- Check if you sit with your back rounded and the hip tilted back. Stretch is reduced on the hamstrings, and high force is created on the discs of the lower back and sometimes the neck. Sitting bent forward, even with a straight back, puts high forces on the back, and is a common contributor to back pain.

Quick Fix:

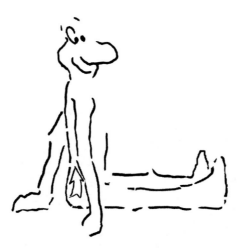

- Put your hands behind you. Push against your hands to lift upward and straighten your back. Using your hands to push up and straighten will increase the stretch and take your weight off the discs of your lower back.

- You will feel the stretch move to your hamstrings right away.

- Sit up straight. Don't round your back, not even a small amount. Lift your chest. You will feel more stretch sitting up straight than leaning forward rounded.

Common Problems in Sitting Hamstring Stretches:

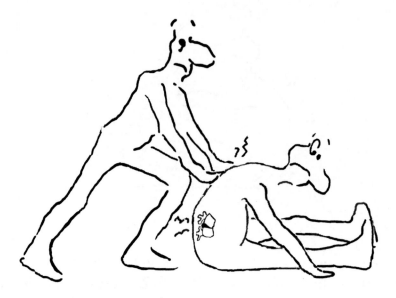

- Sitting, by itself, puts high force on the discs of your lower back. Forcing or pushing someone into a more rounded position while sitting increase forces on the discs.

- Years of sitting and picking things up with rounded back and shoulders, coupled with continued improper stretching, can force the vertebral discs outward, causing degeneration and herniation.

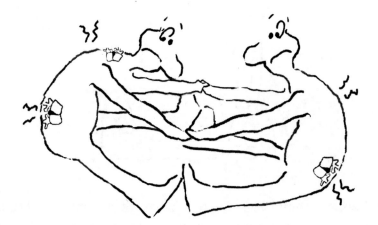

Brain Stretch:

- You know that sitting rounded over a desk, computer, and steering wheel is bad posture. Don't add to bad posture by stretching rounded.

Hamstring Stretch, Lying Down

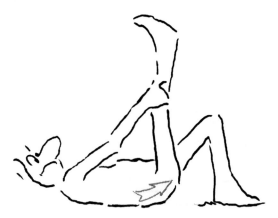

Problem:

- Rounding the back and bending the other leg both reduce the stretch to the hamstrings, and promote rounded posture and tight hips. You also prevent the front of the hip from receiving a much-needed stretch.

Quick Fix:

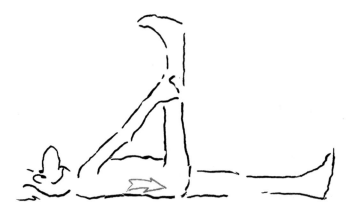

- Lie with your head and shoulders flat, not rounded or lifted upward.

- Keep your hips on the floor, not rounded under.

- Keep the other leg straight, not bent.

- Use your muscles to do the work of holding your back in a healthy position, and feel a healthy stretch in the front of the hip.

Common Problems:

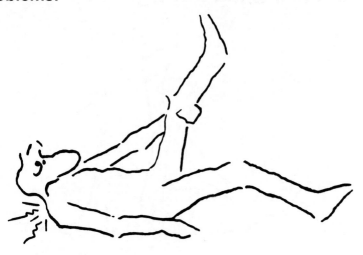

- When you lift one leg to stretch, notice if your other leg pulls upward with it, signaling tight muscles in the front of your hip.

- Notice if your non-stretched leg bends. Instead, hold it flat and straight without locking or forcing.

- Don't lift your head and shoulders from the floor. Rounding your back does not help the stretch in a healthy or effective way, and is unhealthy posture.

Brain Stretch—Use Hamstring Stretches for Healthier Sitting in Daily Life:

- Many people stretch their hamstrings hoping it will help their back. Then they get "mysterious" back pain from unhealthful hamstring stretches.

- The way hamstring stretches help is to allow you to sit without being so tight that your hip curls under you and your back rounds. Tight hamstrings are not as causal in back pain when standing. It's a myth that tight hamstrings would pull your hip forward when standing. If you were that tight, you would not be able to bend enough to sit down without tearing your backside.

- Retrain yourself not to round your back and lean your body weight on your spine when sitting or lifting one leg. Use hamstring stretches to learn and practice holding yourself in healthier spine posture.

Hamstring Stretch, Doorway

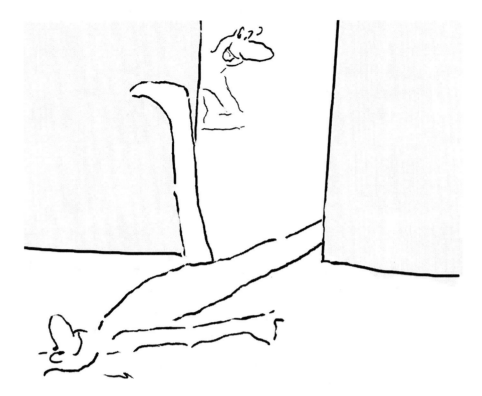

- Lie in a doorway. Lift one leg up to rest against the wall or doorjamb.

- Keep your body, shoulders, and head flat on the floor.

- For more stretch, move your whole body further into the doorway. For less, move away. Relax and breathe. Hold for a few seconds, then switch legs using the other side of the door or wall.

- Keep your hips flat on the floor. Don't let your hips round under you.

- To add stretch for the back of your calf and bottom of your foot, pull your toes back and downward, using your shin muscles or your hand if you can reach.

- A friend can help lift your leg. Remember that the purpose of a stretch is to make things longer and looser. The friend should not push your leg downward toward your body so that the top of your leg bone is compressed into your hip socket. Instead, the friend can allow the hip socket room to stretch by pulling your leg slightly upward and outward while assisting you to stretch your leg.

Hamstring Stretch, Standing and Balancing

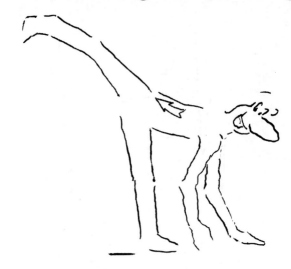

- For a fun, multi-function hamstring stretch, try the "air-split." Keep your back straight and shoulders back, while lifting one leg in back.

- Lean back toward the heel of your standing leg. Don't rock forward toward your toes.

- Keep your body and both hips facing downward, without turning one hip sideways. Keep the standing foot facing straight ahead. Turning sideways reduces or eliminates the stretch on the hamstring.

Common Problems

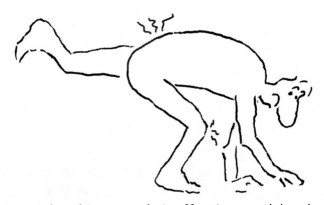

Several bad habits make this stretch ineffective, and hard on your spine and front knee:
- Rounding your back and shoulders forward.

- Leaning your weight toward your toes with your knee forward of your toes. Rocking the knee forward transmits your body weight through your knee joint and takes the exercise off the leg muscles.

- Jutting your chin forward, craning your neck.

Hamstring Stretch Balancing Using a Wall

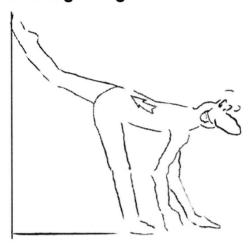

- Stand in front of a wall. Put your hands on the floor and put one leg high against the wall. Lean back toward the heel of your standing leg.

- Keep your back straight and shoulders back. Lift your chest. Don't round your head or chest to your standing leg. Press your lower abdomen toward the leg, while straightening and lengthening the upper body.

- Keep your body and both hips facing downward, without turning to the side. Turning sideways reduces or eliminates the stretch on the hamstring. Keep the standing foot facing straight ahead, not turned out.

Use The Air Split Hamstring Stretch for Healthier Household Bending:

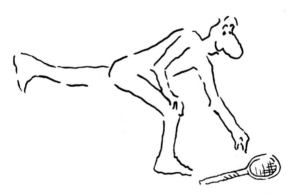

- Raise your back leg as you bend to retrieve objects. Keep your standing heel on the floor with your body weight back toward your heel.

- Keep your back and shoulders straight, not rounded forward.

- Don't jut or push your chin forward.

- Gradually learn to keep the standing leg nearly straight, but not locked straight.

Hamstring Stretch, Balancing Using a Ball

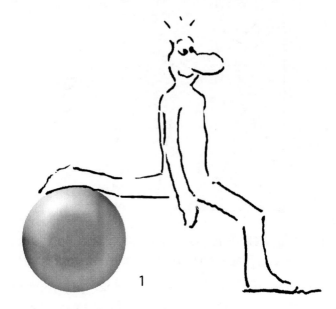

- This stretch has three parts. First, stand with one leg behind you over a ball. Keep your front knee over the heel of your standing foot. You will get good balance practice doing this.

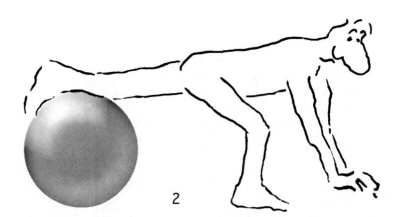

- Next, put your hands on the floor.

- Keep your back straight, your head up, and your shoulders back. If you round your back, you will diminish or eliminate the stretch, and practice bad posture.

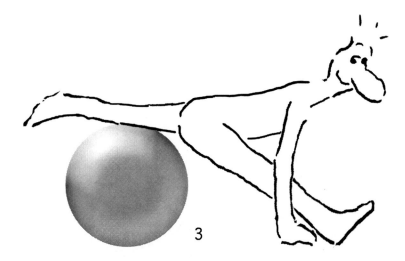

- Push your body backward. Let the ball roll upward to your thigh, above your knee. Progressively straighten your front leg. Keep your back straight, your chest up, and your shoulders back. Keep the rear knee facing downward, not turned out. Smile and breathe.

- Keeping the ball at the thigh, increase the stretch by bending your rear knee so that your foot points upward.

- This stretch can be done with the back leg over various objects at various heights, whether rolling or not. Hold a few seconds and switch legs.

Common Problems:

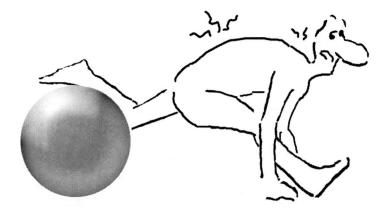

- Rounding your back reduces the stretch on your hamstring, increases force on your discs, and practices unhealthy rounded posture. Craning your neck back and jutting your chin compresses the neck.

- Keep your head up by lifting the chest, not by craning your neck.

Hamstring Stretch, Strength and Balance Using a Wall

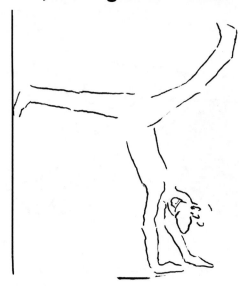

- This stretch does many good things for your body and movement skills at once. It is not as hard as it looks. You may want to avoid this one if you have uncontrolled high blood pressure or problems with pressure in your eyes or brain. Check with your doctor.

- Stand with your back about two or three feet in front of a wall (face away from the wall). Crouch down and put both hands on the floor, as for the hamstring stretch against the wall on page 37.

- Put the bottom of one foot high on the wall. Lift your other leg to the wall. Hold your back straight. Don't let your lower back sag toward the wall, into an arch.

- Don't let your weight pressure your shoulders. Use muscles to maintain shoulder position. Don't let shoulder joints grind under your weight.

- Let one leg stretch overhead away from the wall, as far as you can, to make a split position overhead. To increase the stretch, move the foot that is against the wall down to a lower height against the wall.

- Hold for a few breaths then switch legs to do an overhead "split" on the other side. Keep breathing.

- Holding weight on your arms helps strengthen wrist and arm bones. Strengthening the wrist is important, as the wrist is one of three major sites of osteoporosis. Keep your weight distributed over your entire hand, not concentrated on the wrist, and push with your hand muscles to strengthen without compressing your wrist joints.

- To get back down, bring the stretching leg back to the wall, then step down to the floor gently.

Outside Hip and Side of Body Stretch—Ilio-Tibial Band

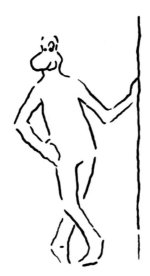

Problem:

- This stretch is commonly done by standing and leaning sideways toward a wall. It is not a bad stretch, just not as effective as other ways to stretch the side of your hip, body, and leg.

Quick Fix:

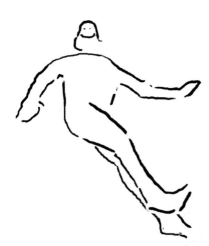

- Lie flat. Bring one leg far to one side. Cross the other leg over it at the ankle so that both legs are far to one side.

- Keep both hips flat on the floor. Don't tilt or lean to the side. Feel the stretch along your side. Keep both legs fairly straight. If you don't feel the stretch, move your legs farther to the side.

- Keep breathing. Hold a few seconds. Breathe in and change sides while breathing out. Repeat on the other side.

Quick Fix #2 for Ilio-Tibial Band Stretch:

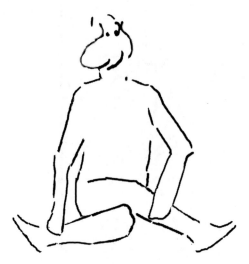

- Sit up straight. Cross one knee over the other knee, touching your knees to each other (or as close as they comfortably reach). Keep both feet far forward of your hips. Your heels should not be near your hips. To move your feet farther away, either push both feet forward with your hands, or slide your behind farther back, away from your feet. You should feel no twisting in your knees. All the stretch comes from both sides of your hips.

- Hold your shins and pull your chest upward and your back straight. You will get more stretch sitting straight than rounding your back.

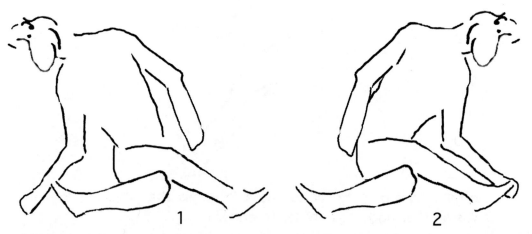

- Gently lean to one side for a few moments (#1 above), then the other side (#2), keeping your legs crossed.

- Cross your legs the other way and stretch to each side again. Keep breathing. Smile.

Anterior Hip Stretch, Standing

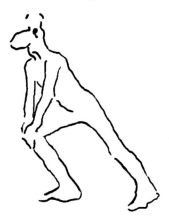

Problem:

- The anterior hip stretch is an important stretch. Unfortunately, it is commonly done in a way that gives little stretch. Leaning forward and turning the back foot outward reduces or eliminates the stretch on the front of the hip (of the back leg). Bringing the front knee forward shifts your body weight to your knee joint and away from your leg muscles, reducing the value of this lunge position as a leg strengthening exercise.

Quick Fix:

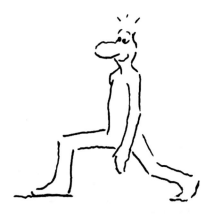

- Turn your back foot completely straight. Don't let your back foot turn outward, not even a small amount. Bend both knees and lift your back heel. Look at your back foot to make sure of straight, not turned-out position.

- Center your body weight between both legs. Take your hands off your front knee.

- Tuck your hip under, as if starting an abdominal crunch, but don't curl forward. Tuck the hip just enough to reduce the low back arch. You will immediately feel the pressure in the lower back stop and the stretch move to your anterior hip muscles (hip flexors) and thigh of the back leg.

Common Problems:

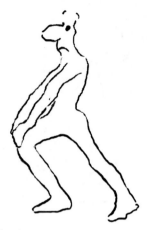

- Arching your lower back.
- Turning your back foot outward.
- Leaning your upper body backward.
- Leaning body weight toward your front knee.

Quick Fix for Anterior Hip Stretch #2—The Lunge:

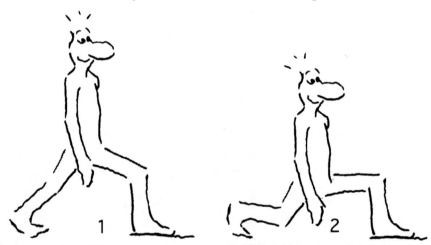

- Start in lunge position, weight centered between both legs (drawing #1 left). Make sure your back foot faces forward, not turned out. Tuck your hip under as if starting an abdominal crunch to reduce the arch in your lower back. Don't round your upper body, just more your hip and spine to neutral.
- Once you feel the stretch move to your hip and thigh, lower straight down to the floor (#2 right). Don't shift your weight to your front knee or let your front knee come forward. Your front knee bends, but does not move forward.

- If your rear knee hurts when standing in lunge or lowering, check that your back leg is far enough back (may need a wider stance), and bent enough, not strained straight. The thigh muscles may be tight and pull on the front of the knee where they attach. Try more anterior thigh and quadriceps stretch, page 9-11.

Brain Stretch:

- The front of your hip is supposed to be able to straighten when you stand, and then extend further when you walk (left drawing below).

- The anterior hip often becomes tight from modern life. Many people sit most of the day, then stand, walk, and exercise with their hip still bent forward (right). The front of their hip tilts forward and downward, increasing the arch in their lower back. They may do stretches for the front of the hip, with the front of the hip still bent forward instead of straightening and extending backward.

- If you stood and moved in a straight healthy manner (left), the front of your hip would get functional stretch throughout the day, and not get tight in the first place.

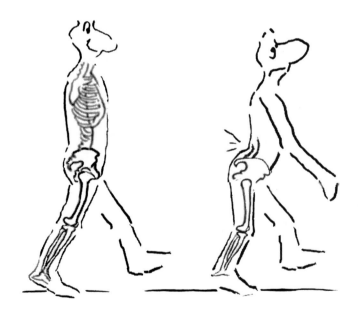

Anterior Hip Stretch, Face Down

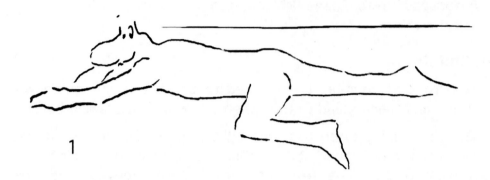

1

- This good-feeling stretch for the front and inside of your hip and leg has four parts. Start by lying face down with one knee bent to one side. Keep both hips facing flat down. To get flatter, push your bent knee further away, out to the side.

- Don't tilt the front of your body toward the bent leg, or you will reduce the stretch. Keep both hips and the inside of your bent leg touching the floor.

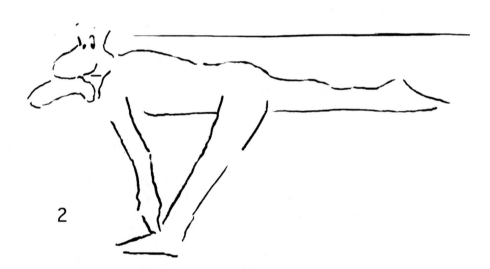

2

- Next, to increase the stretch, straighten your leg to the side, as high as comfortable. Keep both hips flat on the floor. Lie facing flat down, not turned.

- You do not need to touch your hand to your foot to get a good stretch.

- Keep your ankle straight, not bending your foot to the floor.

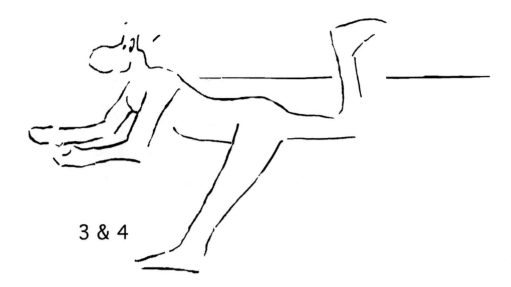

3 & 4

- For the third part of the stretch, prop on your elbows or hands. Don't arch only from your lower back (making it hurt). Instead, gently lift through your entire back, and make sure to get stretch in the front of your hip. To get the most stretch, bend your back knee, so that your foot lifts upward. Smile and keep breathing. Hold the stretch for a few seconds, then repeat the sequence of four stretches with your other leg to the side.

Rocket Ship Face Down

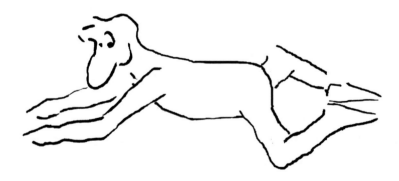

- The Rocket Ship stretch done face down stretches your front (anterior) hip muscles and inside leg muscles at the same time.

- Lie face down. Bring one knee to the side, then the other. Let your feet come off the floor if you are more comfortable that way. Keep your hands anywhere comfortable.

- Relax your shoulders downward. Keep your chin in, not jutting forward.

Anterior Hip Stretch, Face Up

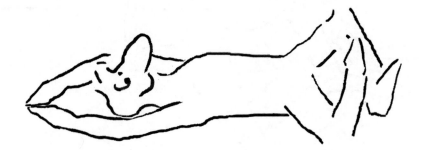

- Several of the stretches for the inside leg also stretch the front (anterior) hip muscles, such as Rocket Ship with legs crossed. Take your shoes off to make room for your feet. Don't cross one leg on top of the other. Let each lower leg rest against the floor.

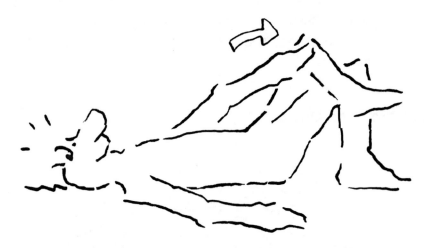

- A nice stretch for the front of the hip starts with a stretch similar to one commonly done for the back of the hip (page 55). Lie face up, crossing one ankle over the other knee.

- Instead of pulling your knee closer to you, push it away with your hand. As soon as you push the knee away, you should feel the stretch move to the front of your hip.

- If you can't reach your knee, put the foot that is on the floor closer to your hip (or you need longer arms).

Anterior Hip Stretch Lying Over a Cushion, Bed, or Ball

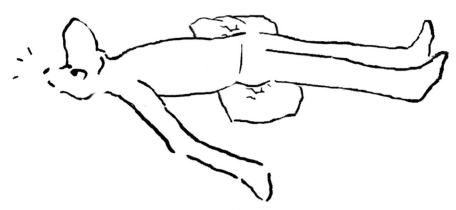

- Lie over a pillow or article of clothing comfortably placed under your hips. Make sure the article is under your behind, not lower back.

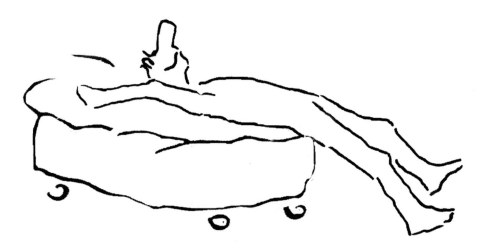

- Lie face up over a bed or bench, with the edge right under your behind. Feel the stretch in the front of your hip.

- Press your lower back toward the bed to avoid arching the lower back. Arching decreases the stretch on the hip and can cause pain.

- To increase the stretch, bring both arms by your ears. You should be able to raise your arms without arching your lower back or feeling pinching in your shoulder. Progress comfortably and intelligently until you can.

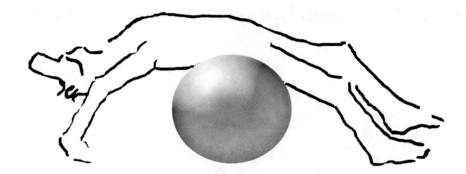

- To stretch your hip over a ball (or other raised object) roll yourself back with arms overhead until the ball is under your hip, not lower back.

- If the backward bending (extension) causes too much pressure in your lower back, tuck your hips to reduce the arch in your lower back, moving the stretch more to the front of your hip.

- To increase the stretch, bring your arms overhead to the floor.

Common Problems:

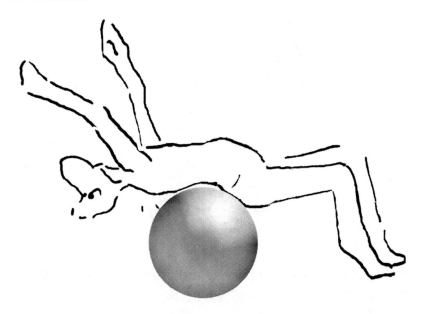

- Putting the ball under your lower back reduces or eliminates the stretch in the front of the hip.

- Keeping the hip bent is the opposite of what you want to achieve by stretching the front of the hip. Straighten your legs to increase the hip stretch.

Anterior Hip Stretch With Lower Back Strengthening

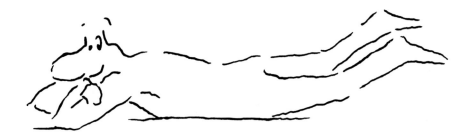

- Lie face down on any comfortable surface. Rest your head and hands any way that you are comfortable.

- Gently lift your legs without bending your knees. Don't force or yank.

- Lift by lengthening the front of your thigh, not by pinching back at your lower back.

- Lift up and down as many times as you can. Start with five or ten and work up from there.

- If lifting both legs at once is too much, start with one leg and increase ability over time.

- If lying face down makes your lower back hurt, it is often the case that the problem is tightness in the front of the hip. Hip tightness makes the lower back arch too much when trying to stand straight or lie flat. Use anterior hip stretches (pages 43-52) to reduce hip tightness, then try lying flat again. Tuck the hip while face down to reduce lumbar spine arch.

- If lying face down makes your thigh hurt down the front, the cause may be tight quadriceps, which cause a tight, pulling sensation. Use the quadriceps stretches (pages 9-10) to reduce tightness, then try lying flat again.

- If lying face down makes your upper back hurt, the reason is often tight front chest muscles, and decreased mobility in the shoulder and upper back. Use pectoral stretches (pages 61-62), anterior shoulders stretches (pages 65-69), the trapezius stretch (page 70), and upper body extension stretches (page 77) to reduce tightness. Then try lying flat again.

Anterior Hip Stretch, Standing With a Ball

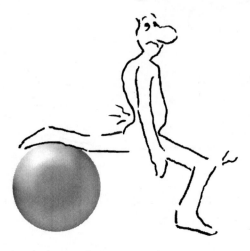

Problem:

- When allowing the lower back to increase in arch, the stretch on the anterior hip of the back leg is reduced. When the front knee is forward of the foot, your weight is shifted more to your knee joint, instead of your leg and hip muscles. When the front heel lifts, stretch on the Achilles tendon and calf muscle is reduced.

Quick Fix:

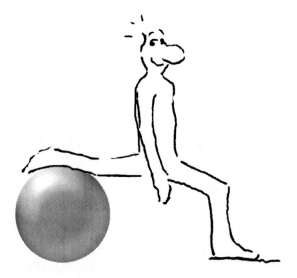

- Tuck your hip under you. You will immediately feel the stretch move to your anterior hip (back leg). Pressure on your lower back will diminish. Tuck as much as you can without rounding your upper body. Don't lean forward or back. Stand straight. Keep your front knee over your heel.

- This stretch can be done with the back leg over various objects at various heights, whether rolling (like the ball) or not.

Posterior Hip Stretch, Sitting

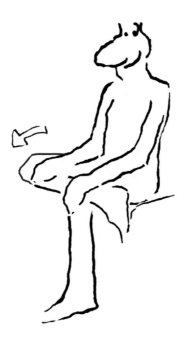

- Sit and cross one ankle over the other knee. Hold your shins and pull yourself up to sit straight.

- Push the crossed knee down and away. The more upright you sit, the more you should feel the stretch.

- Increase the stretch by raising the heel of the foot that is on the floor. Keep pushing the crossed leg down and away.

- Another way to increase the stretch is to lift your chest, keep your back straight, and lean to press your abdomen to your crossed leg. Keep your upper body upright, not leaning over forward. Don't round your upper back in bad posture.

- Try this stretch sitting at a desk with both legs under the desk. When the desk is low enough, you will feel more stretch as you try to keep your crossed leg level under the desk.

Posterior Hip Stretch, Standing

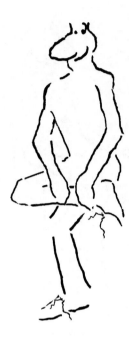

- Stand on one foot. Cross the other ankle over your knee. Bend your standing leg, keeping your body upright and shoulders back.

- It should feel good in the back of your thigh and hip.

- Keep your chin in, not jutting forward. Lift your head up by lifting your chest, not jutting your chin.

- Use this stretch for putting on your socks and shoes every day. You will get a functional stretch, balance, and leg strengthening exercise.

- To improve the stretch and your movement skills, after putting on the first sock, remain standing with your ankle crossed, and bend to retrieve your shoe from the floor. Rise with the shoe, put it on, then change legs for the other sock and shoe.

- To change the stretch and the exercise, lift your knee directly in front of you, not crossed over the other ankle. Hold your knee up and put on your sock and shoe without rounding your back or tilting your head forward. Keep shoulders back, for functional training of posture, balance, and core stability and strength.

- Practice balance safely.

Posterior Hip Stretch, Lying Down

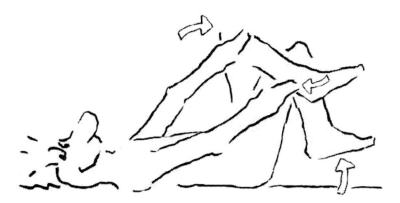

- Lie on your back with one ankle crossed over the other knee. Keep your back, head, and shoulders flat on the floor. (If it is not comfortable for your head and neck to lie flat, try the anterior chest and upper body stretches on pages 61-62 and 77.)

- Slide your foot that is on the floor in the direction of the other foot until you feel stretch on your backside muscles greatly change and increase.

- Push your crossed knee away with your near hand. To increase the stretch, lift the foot from the floor. Keep pressing the crossed knee away with your hand.

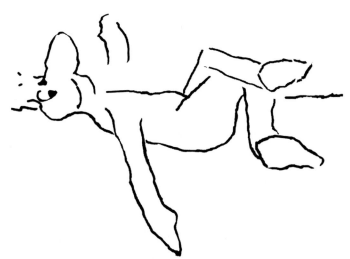

- Gently drop both crossed legs to one side. Hold for a few breaths, then drop to the other side, keeping legs crossed.

- Cross your legs the other way and stretch to both sides again.

- For people who already overdo forward bending, this stretch may increase symptoms of pain in the hip or back. Instead, gently use anterior hip stretches (pages 43-52).

Side Lunge

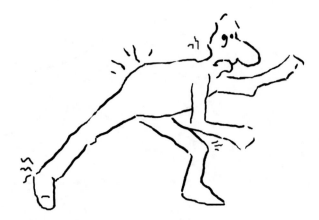

Problem:

- Bending over diminishes stretch in the hip and inside leg muscles, and adds to chronic bending force on the lower back. Leaning the knee forward of the foot shifts weight to the knee joint and off leg muscles. Bending the outside of the ankle may overstretch the side-supporting ligaments, making them loose, increasing chance of ankle sprain.

Quick Fix:

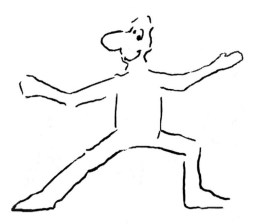

- Keep both heels down flat on the floor. Keep the knee of the bent leg over the heel, not leaning forward of your heel.

- Point each foot outward in the same direction as the knee. Facing the foot in a different direction from the knee, twists the knee.

- Keep your body upright. You will increase stretch on the hips and legs, and overall stretch and exercise for your legs.

Low Side Lunge

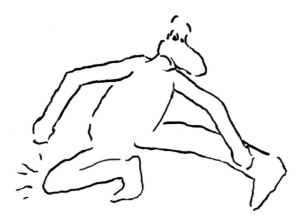

Problem:

- The low lunge stretch is commonly done by squatting on the ball of one foot with the heel lifted. Lifting the heel transfers your weight away from your leg muscles and onto the knee joint, reduces the stretch on the leg and hip muscles of both legs, and eliminates the stretch on the Achilles tendon and calf of the bent leg.

Quick Fix:

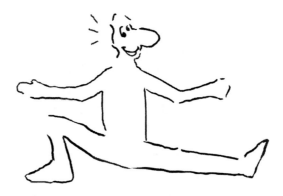

- Keep the heel of your bent leg down on the floor. Keep your knee back over your heel, not forward of your foot. Keep your weight back toward your heel.

- Avoid compressing the bent knee by keeping space between the back of the thigh and calf. Move your foot further away to "open" the space and maintain a larger knee joint angle.

- Turn your other foot so that your toes face upward. Keep the extended leg slightly bent at the knee, not hyperextended backward.

- Keep your body upright.

Lower Back Stretch

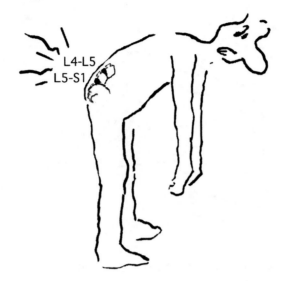

Problem:

- Leaning forward to stretch puts body weight on the discs of the lower back. Forward bending presses the vertebrae together in front, and opens space between them in back. Over years standing bent forward, stretching, sitting, bending, and lifting wrong, the discs between the vertebrae can squash in front and push outward in back, like squeezing a water balloon or tube of toothpaste. This is how discs degenerate and herniate. Disc pain may start suddenly after just one more bend, however, disc injury is usually a gradual process over years, like finally getting chest pain after years of bad eating habits. The discs between your fourth and fifth lumbar vertebrae, and between your last (fifth) lumbar vertebra and your sacrum, usually endure the most weight and pressure from forward bending. That is why the discs herniate most often at these places, abbreviated "L4-L5" and "L5-S1."

- For many people, bending forward to stretch the lower back is not needed or beneficial. Their back is already overstretched and discs overpressured from hours a day of forward bending. Instead, extension help unload the discs and reverse overstretching. Try extension stretches for the upper back, pages 75-77, and hip and lower back on pages 43-52.

- Other people habitually stand, move, and sit with their lower back overly arched. Lower back pain often results from this overarching, also called hyperlordosis. People who overarch usually hurt after walking, jogging, or long standing. They feel they must bend over or lift one leg to relieve it when they should instead, stop overarching. Sometimes, they arch their lower back for so much of the time that the back tightens, and they are not able to stretch their lower spine forward enough to reduce the arch, and stop the pain that comes with it.

Quick Fix #1:

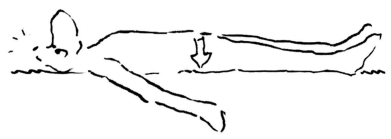

- Lie face up with your legs relaxed straight. Press your lower back downward against the floor or bed. You should feel your hip tilt. This movement is called a "pelvic tilt." If the front of your hip is tight, you may feel your thigh lift from the floor. The purpose of this tilting action is to teach you how to voluntarily reduce an overly large lower back arch. Too much arch causes tightness and pain.

- When you stand up and walk away, use the same tilt to reduce overarching to neutral, and stop back pain. Don't tilt so much that you round forward. The pelvic tilt, done as exercise, does not fix back pain or overarching when standing, but teaches you how to reduce overarching by learning how to hold your spine and hip position when standing. It is not true that you must bend your knees to keep your lower back from arching. You control arching with your torso (core) muscles to tilt your spine into healthy position.

Quick Fix #2 for Lower Back Stretch:

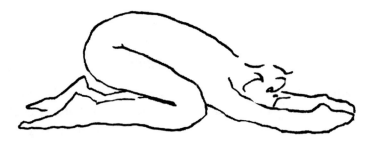

- Occasional rounding stretch is fine, as is the functional slight back stretch of good bending. It is chronic bad daily rounding forward that eventually injures. Kneel with your backside on your heels. Lean forward until your arms and elbows drape on the floor comfortably, either overhead or by your sides. Relax your head down. This stretch is sometimes called "child's pose," because babies and children often sleep this way.

- The discs of your lower back are not usually highly pressured by this bending, because much of your weight is on your arms and thighs, but this stretch, and other lower back stretches are often too much for people with acute disc pain from degeneration, bulging, or herniation.

Foot and Toe Stretches to Straighten Toes

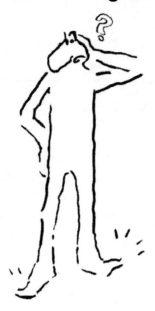

Problem:

- Tight shoes and high heeled shoes can press and deform your toes. Check to see if your toes stick up when you put your foot flat on the floor, or if your big toe tilts toward your other toes on that foot. If your toes fit together like puzzle pieces, your shoes (or socks or stockings) are probably too tight.

Quick Fix:

- Take your toes in your hands everyday, and stretch your toes apart. If toes stick up, stretch them downward. For toes that are shifting toward the other toes, pull them away and straight.

- When you walk, keep both feet facing straight. Don't turn either foot to face outward. Turning out presses the big toe toward the other toes with each step, overstretching the outside of the big toe and promoting "pushed over" toes, hammer toes, and bunion.

- Get out of your shoes and socks every day to stop squeezing and confining your toes. Make sure your feet see daylight for as much time as possible every day for skin and nail health.

- Your toes are important for balance and movement. Toes are not vestigial or useless parts. Make sure you can wiggle and move your toes, and widen them apart from each other.

- For good foot stretches to prevent and reduce the tightness along the bottom that causes plantar fasciitis, try the Achilles tendon stretches on pages 12-17.

Shoulder Stretch, Posterior and Anterior

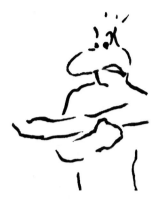

Problem:

- Although the posterior shoulder stretch is one of the most common stretches, it is one of the least necessary. Slouching all day over your desk or while driving over-stretches the back of your shoulders, producing rounded shoulders. Rounded shoulders are a common source of upper back and neck pain. It is unnecessary to further stretch the back of the shoulder.

Quick Fix — Use Anterior Stretches, Not Posterior Stretches:

- The best way to fix rounded shoulders is to skip the posterior shoulder stretch and instead, stretch your chest muscles: Stand facing a wall or in a doorway. Put the inside of one bent elbow against the wall, keeping your elbow level with your shoulder (#1 below). Relax your shoulders. Brace your arm against the wall while turning your feet and body away from the wall (#2). Fee the stretch in your chest, not your shoulder joint. Do this anterior stretch first thing in the morning, and several times during every day to help straighten your posture.

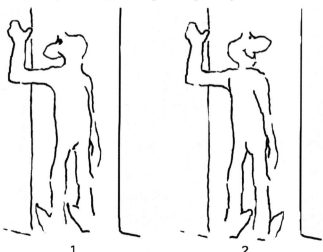

1   2

Quick Fix #2 for Anterior Shoulder Stretch

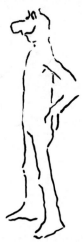

- Put your hands on your hips and bring your shoulders back. You should be able to pull your shoulders back without tilting the front of your shoulders forward or arching your back.

- When you can pull your shoulders back easily with your hands on your hips, try pulling your shoulders back with your hands touching together behind your back, to stretch the front of your shoulder and chest.

Common Problems:

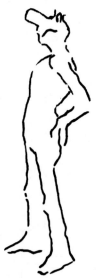

- Letting your shoulders tilt or jut forward.

- Jutting your neck and chin forward.

- Arching your back or leaning back to bring your shoulders back instead of getting the stretch from your front chest muscles.

- Notice any time that you are standing with your hands on your hips, if your shoulders tilt forward.

More Common Problems:

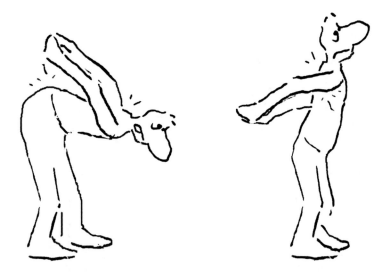

- Turning your thumbs downward moves the stretch away from your front chest (pectoral) muscles where you want the stretch, to your shoulder joint. Moving the stretch to the shoulder joint pushes the top of the arm bone (humerus) into the front of the shoulder joint. The joint space can become compacted, grinding cartilage, and the ligaments that are the "straps" that hold your arm bone to your shoulder can overstretch in front, eventually overstretching until they let your arm bone "rattle" in the joint—rubbing during movement instead of gliding.

- Bending over forward adds degenerating and herniating force on the discs of the lower back.

Anterior Shoulder—Pectoral Stretch With a Partner

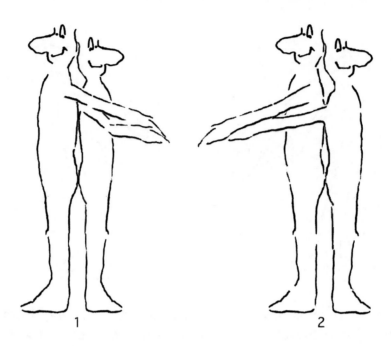

1   2

- Stand back to back with a friend. Stand straight. Touch the back of your hips, upper back, and the back of your head against your partner. Stretch your arms out to the side, thumbs facing upward at about shoulder height. Link hands or arms gently, depending on your relative heights. Elbows stay almost straight, but not locked straight.

- One partner gently pulls arms forward, pulling the other partner's arms backward. The second partner allows the front of the chest to stretch (#1 on left). The stretch does not come from the shoulder joint, but the front chest muscles. Do not bring the shoulder forward, or turn thumbs downward. Don't force. Just stretch. It is supposed to feel good.

- Hold briefly, then switch (#2).

- If you stand bent forward in bad posture, you will push your partner away. Similarly, make sure not to lean back with an overly large inch in your lower back. Don't arch your back to stand straight.

Shoulder and Triceps Reaching Stretch

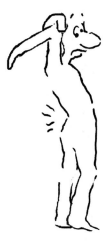

Problem:

- Reaching overhead to pull back the bent elbow is a common shoulder stretch. When it is done with the lower back arched, there is little stretch on the shoulder, but increased pressure on the lower back from the weight of the upper body leaning backward. It is also common to jut the neck and chin forward, practicing bad posture. Most people already overstretch the back of their neck a great deal by slouching over a desk and steering wheel. Adding forward slouching during a stretch is counterproductive to neck health and posture.

Quick Fix:

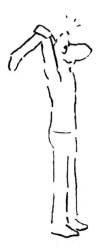

- Tuck your hips under you to reduce the arch in your lower back. Stand straight without pushing your hips forward. You should immediately feel the stretch move to your shoulder and arm.

- Pull your chin in softly, until your head is in line with your body, not forward.

Quick Fix #2 for the Shoulder and Triceps Stretch

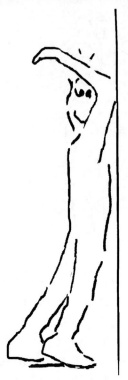

- Place your elbow overhead against a wall. Lean into the wall to press your upraised arm backward.

- Keep your chin in.

- Don't let your lower back arch as you lean. Keep your hip tucked to reduce the lower back arch and keep the stretch coming from the shoulder, not lower back.

- Don't tighten your muscles against the stretch. The purpose of stretching is to lengthen and loosen, not tighten.

Brain Stretch:

- If you are so tight that reaching overhead makes you arch your lower back, you need to stretch the front of your chest and shoulder with the pectoral stretch, pages 61-62, and shoulder stretches on pages 65-70. Sometimes the front of the hip is too tight and limits reaching up. Use the anterior hip stretches on pages 43-52. After stretching so that you are not forced into an arch, you still need to hold your spine position straight so that you don't sag into an arch from sheer lack of using your own muscles to stop it. If your back arches with each overhead reach, imagine the extra strain of the many times you reach to comb, wash, dress, put away groceries, do exercise, and all your daily activities.

Shoulder Stretch Using a Wall

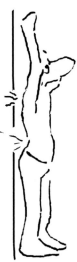

Problem:

- Arching the lower back to raise the arm, reduces or eliminates the stretch on the shoulder, and increases pressure on the lower back. Jutting the head and chin forward or upward practices poor upper body posture, interferes with raising the arm contributing to shoulder pain, and overstretches and strains neck muscles, contributing to neck pain.

Quick Fix:

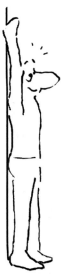

- Keep your hip tucked under to prevent increasing the arch in your lower back. Belt line is level. Feel the stretch come from your shoulder, not lower back.

- Look straight ahead, not jutting your chin forward, up, or down. Keep your head back to leave room in the shoulder for the arm to lift.

- Keep knees straight but not locked back or pressed against the wall.

Shoulder Stretch Lying Down

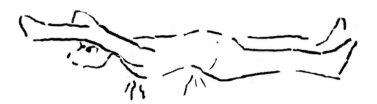

Problem:

- When this lying (supine) shoulder stretch is done by arching the lower back to raise the arm, the shoulder gets little stretch, and pressure increases on the lower back from the arched posture.

Quick Fix:

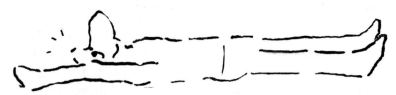

- Keep your hip tucked to prevent increasing the arch in your lower back. Feel the stretch come from your shoulder, not your lower back.

- Keep knees straight but not locked back or forced against the floor.

- Look straight up, not jutting your chin upward.

Brain Stretch:

- Use lying face up as a diagnostic test for tightness in areas that often cause pain during daily life. If you are so tight that you cannot lie comfortably on your back without a pillow under your head, or without your chin jutting upward, you probably need to stretch the front of your chest. Try the pectoral stretch, pages 61-62. If you cannot lie flat comfortably, you cannot stand straight when reaching up during daily activities.

- If it hurts your lower back to lie flat without a pillow under your knees, it is likely that the front of your hip is tight, which forces your lower back to overarch when you straighten your legs. Use the anterior hip stretches on pages 43-52 to restore resting length to the front of your hip. It is not true that you must keep knees bent to protect your back. If that were true, you could never get up and walk away without pain. Stretch wisely so you can stand upright without strain.

Shoulder Stretch Overhead With a Partner

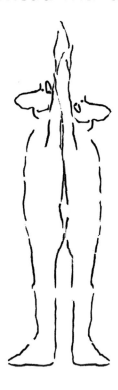

- Stand back to back with a friend. Stand straight Touch hips, upper back, and the back of your head against your partner. Stretch your arms out to the side, thumbs facing upward. Gently link hands or arms, depending on height difference. Elbows stay almost straight, but not locked straight.

- Don't arch your lower back to reach overhead. A small inward curve remains in the lower back, but not a large curve. Stand straight without bending forward or arching backward. Keep your head and neck upright, not tilting or sagging forward.

- Hold arms overhead for a few seconds, breathing normally. Then both partners tilt to one side, arms still touching, pointing like the big hand on a clock to one side. Hold briefly. Breathe in and then breathe out while pointing hands to the other side.

- Use this overhead partner stretch to train straight body positioning, healthy overhead reaching skills, and to get a nice shoulder stretch.

Neck Stretch to the Side—Trapezius

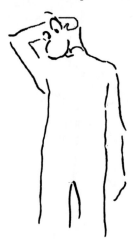

Problem:

- Pulling your head to the side with your hand compresses the neck and spine, and does not give the best stretch for the side of the neck.

Quick Fix:

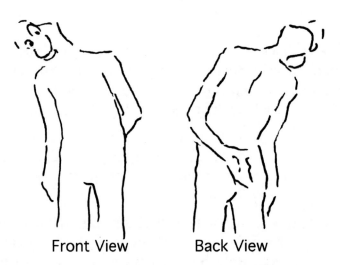

Front View   Back View

- Put one hand behind your back, as if in an opposite pocket.

- Roll your shoulders back and stand up straight. To determine straight position, keep your back and the back of your head against a wall.

- Slide the other hand down your leg toward your knee, gently stretching the entire side of your neck and body. Don't lean your head or body forward. Stand straight.

- Hold for a few seconds. Breathe in, and put the other hand behind you while breathing out to change sides. Repeat on the other side.

Neck Stretch to the Front

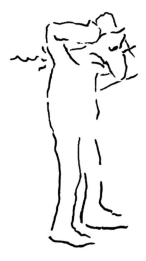

Problem:

- Pulling the head forward to stretch the neck emphasizes and practices the most common bad posture of slouching the head and neck forward.

- Pulling the neck forward compresses the discs and spine. Stretching should make more room, not less.

- Bad forward posture of the head and neck is one of the most common sources of neck pain, upper back pain, and shoulder pain. The forward neck and head is not a posture you want to practice.

More Problems:

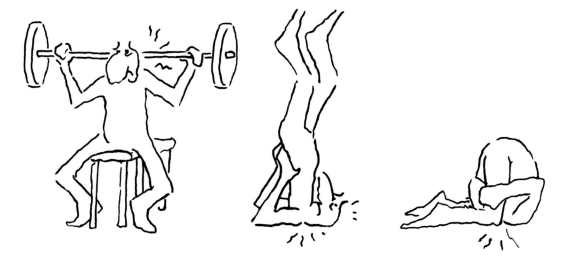

- Forcing your neck forward under the weight of a barbell or your body encourages overstretched forward posture of the neck and compresses the discs. The front of your neck bones pinch together and the space in back opens. Over time, the discs can be squeezed outward, degenerating them, and eventually herniating them. When protruding discs press on nearby nerves, pain can go down your arm with the nerve. Chronically putting pressure on your neck bones can encourage bone spurs to grow.

Quick Fix:

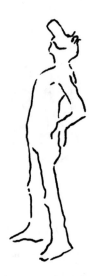

- The best way to fix the bad stretch of pulling your neck forward is to skip it. Instead, stretch backward, not forward, to "unround" your rounded and slouched-forward upper body posture.

- Keep your chin in and shoulders back. Don't arch your lower back to look upward. Let the stretch come from the front of your chest.

Use The Neck Repositioning Stretch for Healthier Daily Life:

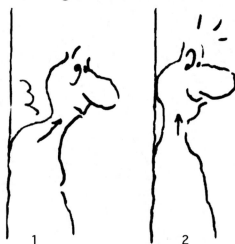

- It is healthy to train your neck away from the forward over-stretched position (#1 above) during your daily activities. Check to see if your head is forward by standing with your back against a wall. Put your heels, your backside, your upper back, and the back of your head against the wall (#2 previous page). That is straight. The common exercise of pulling your chin inward, sometimes called "the double chin exercise," is not something to "do ten times" then walk away with your head forward again. The purpose is to show you where to gently reposition your neck so that you are in healthy position. You only have to do the repositioning one time. Then you hold it. D Don't pull back so hard and far that it makes your neck hurt.

Common Problems:

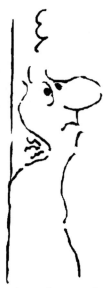

- Jutting your chin upward or forward to bring your head back, or straining to hold straight position. Straight position is not just "ear over shoulder."

Brain Stretch:

- The forward head posture is one of the most common causes of pain in the upper back, shoulders, and neck. The pain is not from stress; but bad posture that you can change. Many people are uncomfortable trying to stand straight because they are so tight that standing straight is a strain. If you have to arch your back and strain your neck to stand against a wall, you are too tight to stand straight. Use the pectoral, triceps, and trapezius, and stretches on pages 61, 66 and 70 to make healthy, straight position easy and comfortable.

- Using the wall to practice straight neck position is not something to do a few times, then go back to slouching forward. Standing against the wall is a test to check positioning. Then you use the information to correct the problem by repositioning your neck and body all the time during all your activities.

Neck Stretch to the Back—Neck Bridge

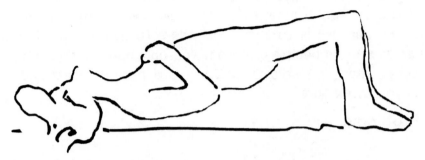

Problem:

- Bridging backward is often used to strengthen and stretch the neck. When the neck is overly craned backward, the spine and soft tissues are compressed, similar to pinching a soda straw.

Quick Fix:

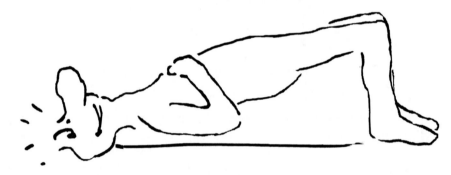

- Keep your neck straight. Bridge on the back of your head, not the top. You will get a better neck strengthening exercise, plus free practice in healthy neck posture for daily life. Skip this stretch (either the bad way or the fix) if you already have a problem with the bad habit of pulling your head back too much or too hard in daily life.

- To advance in strengthening, lift one foot from the floor, keeping your neck straight.

Upper Body Extension Stretch

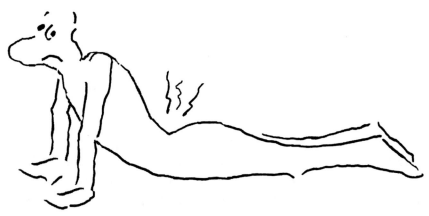

Problem:

- The purpose of this stretch is to "unround" the rounded upper back that occurs with bad posture. Bad rounded posture is a common cause of upper back and neck pain. Often, this extension stretch is done by pinching back from the lower back, never getting the needed stretch in the rest of the spine. Hyperextending your elbows (letting them bend backward) under your weight is another common problem that can eventually wear on your elbow joints.

Quick Fix:

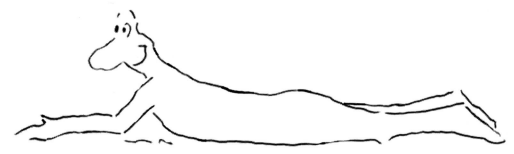

- Prop on your elbows, hands facing down. Without moving your hands, press them down against the floor and pull your hands and elbows strongly against the floor toward your chest. Push your abdomen down against the floor. Feel the pressure move away from your lower back, and the stretch move to your upper back.

- Don't lift up by only pinching your lower spine backward. Get the stretch throughout your upper back.

- Use this upper body extension stretch first thing in the morning before getting out of bed, instead of sitting on the bed, to practice starting the day straight. Use this stretch to "unround" your back and unload your discs after sitting and working bent over.

Upper Body Extension for Strengthening

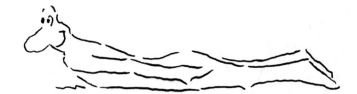

- Upper back extension does three important things that help stop back pain. Stretching backward "unrounds" bad, rounded upper back posture. Extension unloads the discs that are loaded by forward bending. Contracting the upper back muscles strengthens the muscles you use to keep your upper body from slouching and rounding forward.

- Lie face down on any comfortable surface. Gently lift your upper body without using your hands. Don't force or yank. Keep your chin in, not jutting forward. Don't force or yank. Lift up and down as many times as you can. Start with at least five or ten and work up from there.

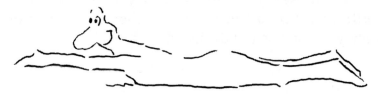

- As you progress, lift your hands in front of you to add more weight and exercise.

- Lift easily, getting the stretch along your entire back, not just "folding" your lower back.

Brain Stretch:

- The purpose of upper body extension is to make it comfortable to stand straight instead of rounding forward. Body positioning is not automatic just with stretching. The stretch makes it possible, but you are the one to hold good posture. After doing stretches, remember to stand straight.

- Many people stand and move in much of the day letting their lower back arch backward too much (hyperlordosis). Overarching in hyperlordosis exaggerates the normal inward curve. Hyperlordosis (overarching) is one major, and often missed, cause of pain and pressure in the lower back. The purpose of extension exercises is not to add to forced arching in the lower back. The purpose is to contract the upper back muscles to strengthen them, and get a gentle extension stretch along the entire spine, while learning to not fold the lower back under your weight.

Upper Back and Chest Stretch Over a Pillow Or Bed

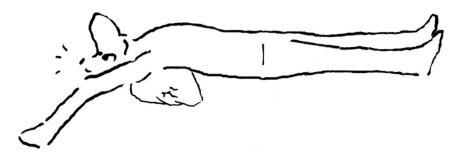

- Lie over a pillow or article of clothing comfortably placed cross-wise under your upper back. Don't put the pillow under your head or neck.

- Let your upper back extend backward. Notice the feeling of the upper back no longer rounded forward.

- To increase the stretch, bring both arms by your ears. You should be able to raise your arms without arching your lower back or feeling pinching in the shoulder.

- For another pillow stretch to help unround your shoulders, lie on your back over a narrow roll or rolled towel lengthwise from the back of your head down the middle of your upper back. Let your shoulders relax backward and down to the floor (or bed).

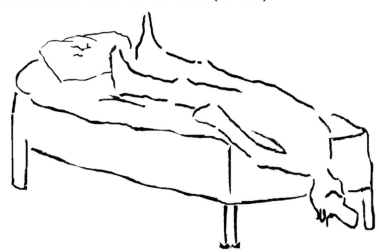

- Lie backward over the soft edge of a bed or bench. Place the edge right under the middle of your upper back, where you need to "unround" the most.

- Don't let your neck bend pinch backward; hold your neck straight. Raise your hands by your ears to increase the stretch.

Stretching Breaks for Travelers

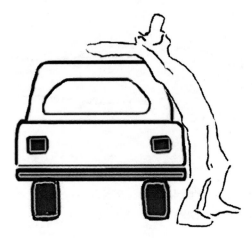

- Take breaks to stand up from long sitting on road trips. Even if you sit with good positioning, sitting is a lot of forward bending, which loads the discs and soft tissue of your back, and shortens and tightens the muscles in front of your body.

- Stand with your back against the side, hood, trunk, or other sturdy part of the vehicle, or safe object. Lean back comfortably. Bring both arms overhead by your ears to increase the stretch. You should be able to raise your arms without your lower back being pulled into an uncomfortable arch, or feeling pinching in your shoulder.

- While seated, keep a small towel or soft roll between the "small" of your lower back and the seat back to help you sit with a slight inward lower back curve. If the roll does not feel comfortable, it is usually too large, made of materials that are too hard, or you may not have placed it comfortably.

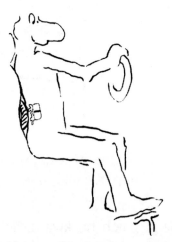

- Test the comfort and size of a lumbar support by putting your hand or forearm between your lower back and the seat back. Do not round against your hand or push your lower back against your hand. Sit up and lean back, pressing your upper body back, not your lower back. Feel how and where you can sit comfortably straight using your hand or forearm as a lumbar roll, then make your lumbar roll the same size and placement. A lumbar roll can be any small comfortable article of clothing, towel, rag, toy, foam roll, a pair of gloves, the sleeves of a jacket, or a commercially purchased soft form.

- If you are driving, before putting the vehicle in motion, test how it feels to slide your seat forward and tilt the seat back slightly backward. Then you can reach the wheel or controls without leaning forward and rounding your back. While driving, check your shoulders often to see if you are holding them tightly or hunching them upward. Stretch your shoulders down and back. Check if you are tightening or rounding your back or neck forward. Breathe and relax them downward. Make sure they can move and wiggle freely.

- Take a big yawn now and then to stretch your lungs. Mixing bigger sighs with normal breaths helps lung function.

- Airplane and bus seats are sometimes so rounded that you need two lumbar rolls. Put one to pad the space between your lower back and the seat, and another above it behind your upper back so that you can sit up and lean back, instead of rounding your back to fit the rounded seat.

- Stretching recommendations for long air flights sometimes list bending forward at the neck, waist, or hips. After long sitting, you do not need more forward stretching. If you are a passenger in an airplane flight or other vehicle, stretch your neck and shoulders to the back instead of only forward. Twist in your seat to each side to brace your elbow against the seat back for the pectoral stretch (page 61). Stretch the back of your legs by straightening your knees and pulling your toes back with your shin muscles. Increase leg circulation by pressing both feet against each other, then cross your ankles and pull both feet outward against each other, then cross your ankles the other way and repeat. When you have the opportunity to get out of your seat, stretch to restore length to the front of your hip with lunges (page 44), quadriceps stretches, (page 9) and others that you enjoy. It is easy and unobtrusive to do wall stretches while waiting for the rest room (pages 67, 81-83).

Side and Upper Body Stretch

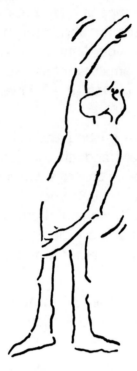

Problem:

- This common stretch does little to stretch anything.

Quick Fix:

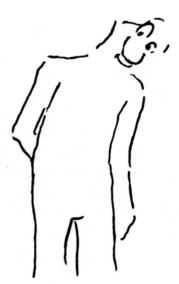

- To increase the stretch on the side of your neck and body, put one hand behind your back, as if in an opposite pocket. Slide the other hand down the side of your body.

- Keep your shoulder rolled back and your head and upper body from tilting or leaning forward.

- To practice straight positioning, do this stretch with your back and the back of your head against a wall. Don't let your head or upper body come forward of the wall as your stretch to the side.

- Gentle leaning side to side helps push nutrients in and wastes out of your vertebral discs. Joints and discs need movement for health.

Quick Fix #2

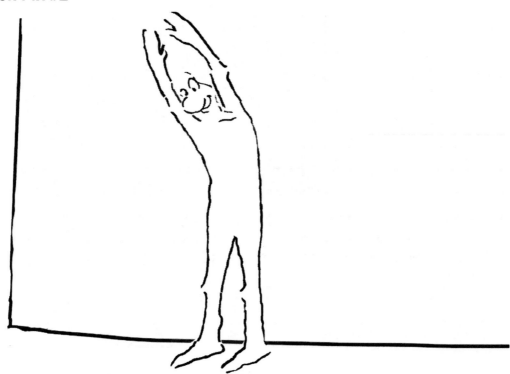

- Stand with your back against a wall. Touch your heels, backside, upper back, the back of your head, and both hands overhead, against the wall. Keep your fingers touching the wall while you stretch to one side. Hold briefly, breathe in, and then stretch to the other side while breathing out.

- Keep your heels, hip, upper back, back of the head, and fingers touching the wall. Don't force the back of your knees against the wall; allow a space. A small space also remains between your lower back and the wall, but not a large space.

- Notice if you arch your lower back more when you reach up to touch the wall. Don't allow your lower back to increase in arch. Get the stretch from your shoulders, not by arching your back or leaning back.

Wrist and Forearm

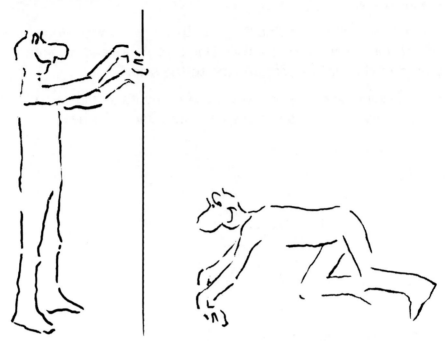

- Face a wall or kneel with both palms up, as if offering a bowl. Point your fingers downward and press your palms against the wall or floor.

- Increase the stretch by placing your hands higher on the wall, or farther away on the floor. Bend your elbows more to get more stretch. Don't lock your elbows straight, or hyperextend your elbows backward.

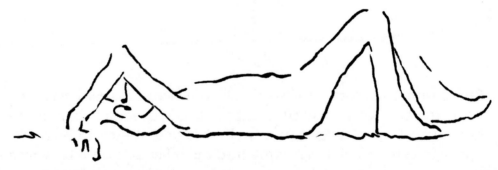

- A nice combination wrist and shoulder stretch starts with lying face up. Bring both arms overhead (or one arm if that works better), with fingers pointing back to your shoulder. Keep hands facing as straight as possible without turning them out.

- Lying face up is the same position you can use to push up into a back bend. Push up safely, getting the stretch along your entire back, not just pinching and tightening one area. When coming back down, make sure not to land on your head.

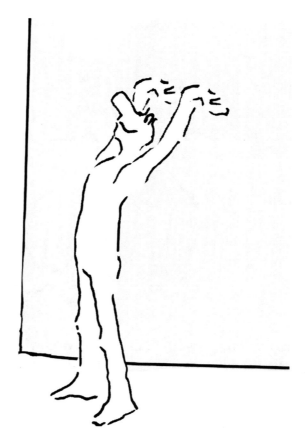

- For a nice combination arm and body stretch, stand with your back about a foot or two in front of a wall.

- Reach overhead to touch your fingers to the wall, fingers pointing downward and palms upward.

- Press your palms to the wall, straightening your elbows as much as feels good. Don't lock your elbows straight or hyperextend your elbows backward.

- Lift upward in your chest to keep your body weight from pressing downward on your lower back. Don't pinch your lower back under your weight. Keep lifting upward gently. Keep breathing.

- To increase stretch, strength, and balance component, "walk" your hands down the wall toward the floor, then "walk" back up to a standing position. Keep lifting upward strongly, using your abdominal muscles, to keep your weight from pressing downward on your lower back.

- Retrain healthy use of your wrists by keeping your weight distributed over your hand and arm muscles, not mashing your wrist joints backward. Whenever you press weight on your hands to prepare food, type, drive, wring clothing, exercise, or stretch, use arms and hand muscles, instead of allowing the move to compress or twist the wrist joints.

Face Stretch

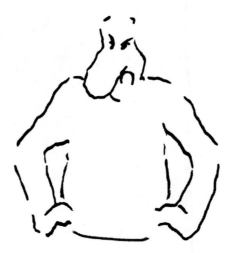

Problem:

- Frowning stretches your face in the wrong direction for mood and social interaction, and does not work the muscles that keep your face looking healthy and uplifted.

Quick Fix:

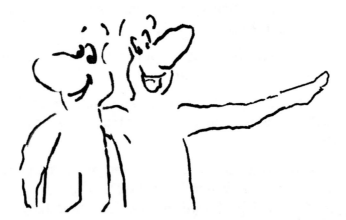

- Smile. Use your facial muscles to lift your spirits, health, and appearance. Use facial and body muscles to laugh, and improve frame of mind, circulation, lung function, and other health aspects.

- When you do this happy face stretch with genuineness, you stretch yourself plus other people. Positive responses can continue from person to person, to workplaces, to countries, to worlds. Give it a try.

- Enjoy your stretching.

Stretches That Make You Tighter

Problem:

- People often work hard and strain to achieve a range of motion in the name of stretching. Stretching in tight, forced, strained ways can stress ligaments (joint attachments), destabilize joints, strain joint capsules enough to injure them, and not surprisingly, tighten muscles.

Problem #2:

- Many people hunch and bend forward over their computers, desks, and steering wheels. Over time, their back muscles become overly rounded and elongated while their front muscles become short and increasingly tight, contributing to round-shouldered and bent-hipped posture.

- Many common stretches contribute to postural tightness. Many people do most of their stretches by bending forward. They touch toes by bending forward, bring knees to chest, chin to chest, bring the arm forward over the body, lunge forward, hang forward at the waist, and other forward bending stretches. Habitual rounding causes problems in the muscles, bones, and discs of your neck and back.

- The result is that the average person is too tight to even stand up straight. This tightness often results in needless pain from chronic low-grade aches, injury, decreased range of motion, and wear and tear from habitual unhealthy positioning.

Brain Stretch:

- The best use of stretching is to restore healthy muscle length to keep your joints in healthy position and to retrain relaxed movement.

- Many people, including some who can touch their toes and bring their foot behind their head, are often too tight to just stand up straight.

- See if you stand straight by trying the following posture test. Stand with your back near a wall. Back up until something touches the wall. See if your hips touch first or if your upper body touches first.

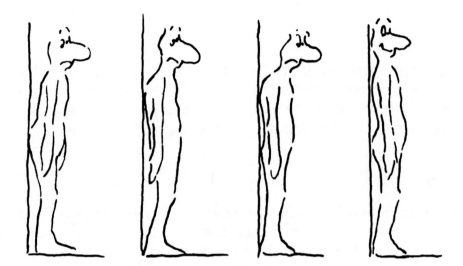

- If you touched your hips to the wall first (left), you may stand bent forward at the hip because of anterior hip tightness. Use the anterior hip stretches on pages 43-52. Then try the wall posture test again and feel the difference in ease of standing.

- If you touched your upper back to the wall first (second from left), you may arch you back too much, and need to practice standing straighter without letting your hip sag forward and your upper body backward. Try the hip tilt at the top of page 59 to learn how to reduce an overly large lower back arch.

- Now stand against the wall touching your heels, hips, and upper back. If it is uncomfortable to bring the back of your head against the wall (second from right), your anterior chest and shoulder may be too tight. Use the pectoral stretch, pages 61-62 and the trapezius stretch, page 70. Then try the wall posture test again and feel the difference in ease of standing.

- If it hurts your lower back to bring your head back against the wall, you are probably arching your back. The front of your hip may be too tight to allow you to extend straight. The lower back compensates by arching. Use the anterior hip stretches, pages 43-52.

- Use all the needed stretches so that straight standing is normal and comfortable. You should notice a difference as soon as you do the stretches and try the wall posture test again. Whenever you pass a wall or doorway or stand in an elevator, see if you can touch your hips, upper back, and the back of your head easily and comfortably against the wall (right drawing). Then hold the healthy, comfortable, straight position when you walk away from the wall. Instead of straining and tightening to stand straight, you will be able to stay relaxed and straight.

Overstretching Bad Habits In Daily Life

Problem:

- It's not true that most people never stretch. Many people stretch a great deal every day during daily activities by letting their body slouch. Slouching is a stretch, just not a beneficial one. Check yourself for simple bad habits.

Overstretching Your Neck Forward

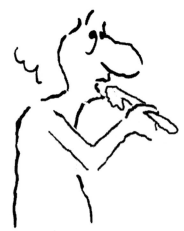

- Letting your head and neck sag forward is called a "forward head." The forward head is a common cause of pain in the upper back, neck, and across the shoulders.

- Over time, the back of the neck overstretches and the front of the neck and chest shortens and tightens. Soon, the tightening in front makes it too uncomfortable for you to stand straight, in a cycle of pain and tightening.

- Holding your neck forward reduces or eliminates the normal small inward curve (normal small lordosis). Shock absorption is reduced, pressure increases on the discs, and space opens at the back of the vertebrae. Over years, the discs of the neck can degenerate and be pushed outward, (herniate).

- Notice your head and neck position during daily activities. Use the pectoral and trapezius stretches on pages 61-62 and 70, and the upper chest stretches on pages 75-77, to restore resting length to the chest and top of the shoulder and neck so that you can stand with healthy head and neck position.

Craning Your Neck

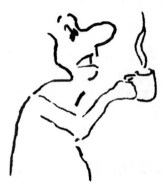

- Check if you jut your chin forward and pinch the neck back when looking and reaching upward, drinking, using binoculars, and other upward-gazing activities. Craning makes a postural spondylolisthesis, pushing vertebrae and discs forward of the ones below. Scary on x-rays but not a disease, just a bad posture.

- To lift your face upward, lift your chest instead of pinching your neck backward. Keep chin in, not jutting forward. Don't arch your lower back to look upward, but lift from the upper body, unrounding the upper back. You will get a built-in upper body stretch, stop pain from neck craning, and help prevent round-shoulders and neck pain.

Sitting With Your Back Rounded

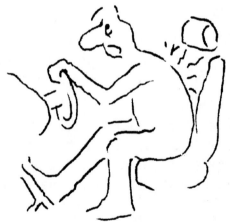

- Sitting with your back rounded over your computer or steering wheel is a common cause of upper and lower back pain. Your back overstretches and the front of your chest shortens and tightens.

- Over time, the tightening in the front muscles of your chest makes it too uncomfortable for you to sit with your upper body straight instead of rounded, in a cycle of pain and tightening.

- Notice your upper body position during all sitting. Use the pectoral and trapezius stretches on pages 61-62 and 70, and the upper chest stretches on pages 75-77 to restore resting length to upper body so that you can sit with healthy upper body position.

- Move your car and desk seat in to sit closer, so you can sit up and back, instead of rounding forward.

Bending With Your Back Rounded

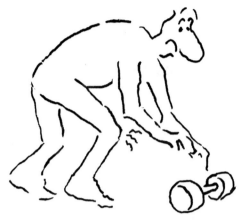

- Bending with injurious body mechanics (bending wrong) is a common cause of lower back pain. Notice your body position during all the many times you bend during daily life and exercise. Keeping your back straight is not enough to prevent back injury if you bend over and lift with straight legs, as high leverage still falls on your back.

- Keep your back upright. Bend your knees, keeping your knees over your heels with your weight back toward your heels, not leaning forward. Use the lunges on page 43 for practice. Bend right for all lifting, whether for packages, cleaning, or picking up weights in the gym. It's free leg exercise.

Standing With Your Upper Back Overly-Rounded

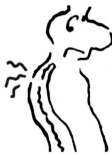

- Letting your upper body sag and round forward is a common cause of upper back pain, and pain across the back of the shoulders.

- Over time, the upper back overstretches and the front of the chest shortens and tightens. The tightening in front can make it too uncomfortable to stand with your upper body straight instead of rounding forward, in a cycle of pain and tightening.

- Notice your upper body during daily activities. Use the pectoral and trapezius stretches on pages 61-62 and 70, and the upper chest stretches on pages 75-77, to restore resting length to the muscles in your chest and top of the shoulder and neck, so that you can stand with healthy upper back position.

Exercising With Your Back Rounded

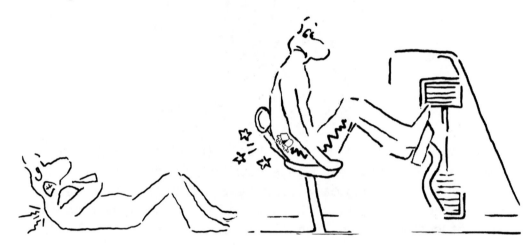

- Many people round over their desk all day then exercise with more forward rounding. The back and shoulders become overstretched. Chronically holding a muscle in a stretched position weakens it. The characteristic "round-shouldered" posture that can result is often clinically identified as a "stretch-weakness."

- People with disc pain and osteoporosis are at even higher risk of injury from forward bending exercises.

- Instead of forward rounding, stand for leg press exercises to get functional strengthening that transfers to how you need your legs in real life. Use extension stretches and exercises on pages 75-77. Instead of crunches, try "The Ab Revolution™" which is a system of core strengthening without forward bending. See the resource list on page 106.

Reclining With Your Back Rounded

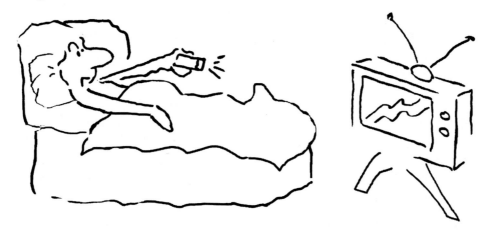

- It is common to read and watch television in bed with the spine rounded forward on pillows, pressuring the back and practicing rounded posture that can make daily life tight and uncomfortable.

- Instead of putting pillows only under your head and upper back, put one (or more as needed) under your lower back to preserve the natural small inward curve of the lower back, and help prop you up without strain and rounding in your upper body.

Standing With Your Lower Back Overly Arched

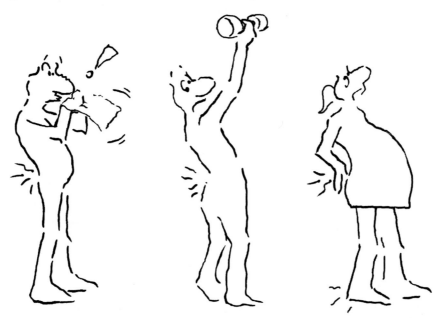

- Arching your lower back by leaning back with your hip pushed forward (left) or stuck out in back (middle and right) is a common source of lower back pain. This over-arching (hyperlordosis) is not unchangeable anatomy or desirable posture. It is bad posture.

- When carrying any load in front, from groceries, to a chair, to a pregnancy, or a baby on your hip, don't lean back to offset the load. Stand straight.

- To stop the arching and the lower back pain that results, tuck your hips under you as if starting an abdominal crunch. Don't over-tuck, round your shoulders, or lean forward or backward. Just stand straight. When you tuck properly by moving your spine (not by tightening anything) the too-large arch will lessen to normal, and pressure in your lower back from the arching should immediately disappear.

- If you habitually stand with your lower back arched, it can eventually tighten, making it hard for you to stand, or even lie down, without arching and lower back pain. Becoming tightened into an arch can also predispose you to muscle spasm or pain when doing the important back extension exercises. Use the lower back stretches on page 59.

Exercising With Your Lower Back Overly Arched

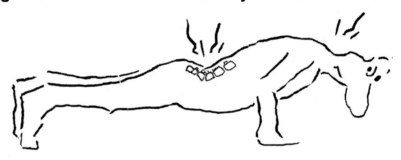

- Pushups are often done for "core" exercise. When done with the lower back arched, body weight shifts to your spine, reducing, or more commonly, eliminating the exercise on abdominal and core muscles.

- When holding a pushup position, tuck your hip as if starting an abdominal "crunch" to straighten your spine. When you rotate your hip (tuck your tailbone) to straight position and reduce the too-large lower back arch, you will immediately feel the effort shift to your abdominal muscles. The pressure and overstretching in the lower back will stop.

- Hold your head up, not sagging downward. Keep your neck straight to practice using your muscles to hold neck position in the way you need for healthy standing.

Standing Bent Forward at the Hip

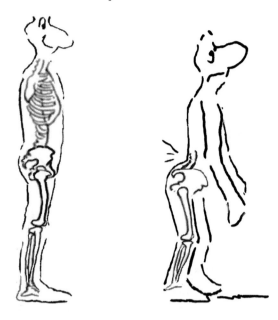

- It is common to sit much of the day with the hip bent, then stand and move with the hip still bent. Keeping muscles bent tightens them.

- Walking and moving bent at the hip puts the muscles of the hip and back of the leg, and gluteal (backside) muscles in a state of reduced use, altering gait, and reducing muscle use and exercise.

- Notice if you can keep your hip and body straight when raising one leg high to stretch, step up, dance, or kick. If the leg you are standing on pulls forward as your raise the other leg, the front of your hip may be tight.

- Use the anterior hip stretches on pages 43-52 to restore resting length to make healthy straight standing comfortable. Then hold relaxed, comfortably straight positioning for standing activities. It is sometimes asked if it is "normal" to be tighter in the front muscles than the posterior muscles. You should not be so tight that you stand bent. It may be normal to wet your pants too, but you learn healthy control.

- Notice if you are bending forward when you could be standing upright. Check your positioning over counters, crutches, walkers, workbenches, household chores, vacuum cleaners, babies, and sinks. For bending, bend your knees, keeping your weight back toward your heels, and your upper body upright.

Reclining Bent Forward

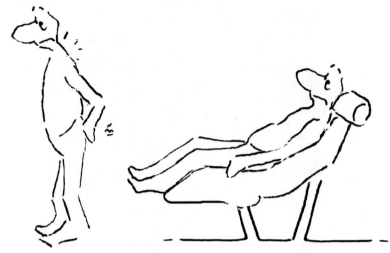

- Chairs are often designed by having representative models sit "comfortably." Often "comfortably" meant "bad rounded posture" because the models were too tight to sit straighter without strain.

- Check recliners, chaise longue, patio furniture, "zero-gravity" chairs, salon and dental chairs, and adjustable beds for backs and headrests that promote forward head, rounded lower back, and rounded upper back.

- Avoid sleeping regularly in chairs or beds that keep you bent forward at the back, neck, hip, and knee. You may overstretch your muscles and joints in back and tighten in front until you become unable to stand or rest comfortably without being bent forward in the same way. Then you will add to pain, not reduce it.

Side Hip Slouching

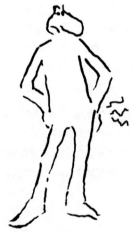

- Stretching the side of your hip is nice. Routinely standing and walking with your weight shifted to the side pressures the hip socket, contributing to hip pain.

- Notice when walking or going up and down the stairs if you shift your weight sideways as you step. Hold yourself level using your hip and leg muscles.

Knee Hyperextension

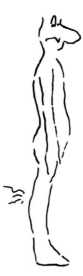

- Habitually standing with your knees "locked" and pressed backward overstretches and pressures the knee joint, contributing to knee pain.

- When standing and walking, notice if you push your knees backward, or if you "rest" by locking your knee joint. Instead, keep your weight on your leg muscles, without locking your knees straight or pushing your knees backward.

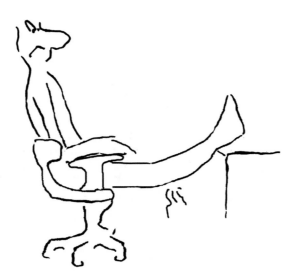

- Sitting with your knees hyperextended for long periods can gradually overstretch the knee and make it hurt.

"Duck-Foot"

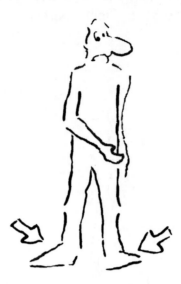

- Walking with your feet turned out pressures the inside of your ankle and knee, and flattens your arch. Standing and walking with your feet turned outward loses the natural stretch along your Achilles tendon and bottom of your foot (plantar fascia). Pulls and pain can result.

- You can eventually become so tight that it feels uncomfortable or "unnatural" to walk with both feet pointing straight ahead.

- Keep both feet and both knees facing forward when standing, walking, and moving, for built-in, natural, healthy stretch. Use Achilles tendon stretches on pages 12-17.

Round Shoulders

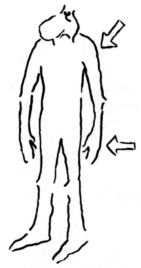

- Letting your shoulders and upper back round forward can eventually overstretch and weaken your upper back, and tighten your chest and shoulders so much that your can feel unnatural or strained to stand straight.

- When your shoulders round, your arms rotate inward. To check for this rotation, look down at your hands when you are standing comfortably, and see if your thumbs face each other instead of facing straight forward. If your hands turn inward, use the pectoral stretch on page 61-62 to restore resting length to your front chest muscles.

Outside of the Ankle

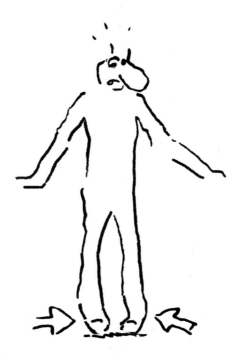

- When standing on tiptoe, don't let your weight teeter outward over your little toes, bending the side of the ankle.

- The tough "straps" (ligaments) that hold your leg bones to your ankle bones are not supposed to stretch much. They are supposed to stay at the length that keeps you from turning your ankle sideways, spraining it.

- When you overstretch your ankles with bad stretches (top of page 27) and through daily bad habits, you may increase your risk of sprains.

- Practice standing on your toes, keeping your body weight over your big toe and second toe. Don't let your ankles sag inward or outward; hold your ankles straight. Then practice rising up and down, keeping your ankles straight. Work up rising to toe on one foot, then to careful jumps, first on both feet, then on one foot, coming down with your weight centered over your big and second toe, not turning your ankle outward.

With this practice, you can train your ankles to deliberately hold healthy position with each foot-fall, reducing your risk of sprains.

- Shoes are not supposed to be tight. "Support" to hold your ankle position can, and should, come from your own foot, ankle, and leg muscles. Healthy ankle and foot posture is no different than holding good upper body posture by not letting your head and shoulders sag and slouch forward.

Inside of the Ankle

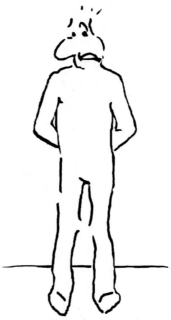

- You can hold ankle and foot position so that you have healthy arches, or you can let your arches flatten under your body weight.

- Your ankles and legs have posture, the same as your shoulders and back. You control that posture with your own muscles and brain.

- When standing, don't let your weight fall inward, bending your ankle inward and flattening your arches.

- Keep your weight distributed over the sole of your foot, instead of leaning inward on your arches. You will use muscles on the outside of your legs and ankles.

- Holding your ankles straight for standing and walking is no different than a beginning skater, who at first sags and tilts inward, then learns to hold their ankles straight.

Fun Flexibility Facts

Is Stiffness Unavoidable With Aging?

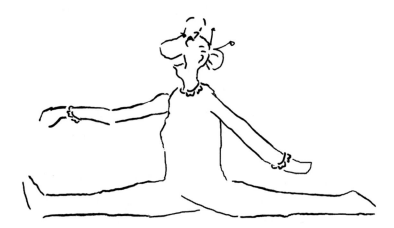

- Getting stiffer with disuse is often confused for aging. If you pass time without stretching, you will get tighter whether you are younger or older. Stretching is like other skills. Practice regularly in the right way and you will get better. After 20 years of studying a foreign language, for example, you probably will be more advanced than you are now. If you stretch well for the next twenty years, you can be more flexible than you are now, and move with ease. Make sure to exercise too, not just stretch. Exercise improves strength, circulation, general health, joint health, and generates anti-inflammatory chemicals. You can regain the functional abilities of chronologically younger person. Stretching a few times a week or before an activity will not reverse daily bad movement habits and tightening, so stretch a few moments each day and also move with healthy body mechanics throughout the day. Build functional stretches into everyday life and you can avoid getting tight in the first place.

What Does "Double-Jointed" Mean?

- "Double-jointed" is an expression meaning to have good flexibility. It is only an expression. Some people may have joints that allow more motion due to the shape of the joint or looseness of the structures that hold the joint together. There are no actual doubled or duplicate joints that increase flexibility.

Does Being Muscular Make You Tighter?

- Strengthening your muscles does not decrease flexibility. Lack of stretching makes you tighter. Exercising for strength can increase muscle density, fiber, and water content, making the muscle (and you) firmer. Exercising should not result in "tightening" the muscle or holding it with extra tension. You cannot move properly when you hold your muscles tightly. Increased muscle firmness is sometimes called "tight," but holding your body tightly is a bad tension habit, not a result of strengthening.

Do You Have to Warm Up Completely Before All Stretching?

- Increasing your body temperature increases flexibility. You don't need to bicycle or jog for 10 minutes to become warm. A few pushups and lunges will have you breaking a light sweat and increasing whole body circulation within seconds. Hot showers, tubs, steams, and saunas can also help.

- For many of the stretches in this book, for example, to stretch the front of your chest and hip to restore healthy posture, you do not need to sweat. Restoring functional muscle length should not be so strained that tears occur in muscles that are not warmed above resting temperature.

What is Reciprocal Inhibition?

- "Reciprocal inhibition" refers to the assumption that if you contract a muscle, the opposite muscle (the reciprocal muscle also called antagonist) will automatically be inhibited making it relax and stretch. However, several things prevent this from working as hoped. Many people strain and tighten muscles on all sides of the area because of bad stretching habits, trying too hard, or just uncoordinated efforts. The reciprocal muscles never loosen. Other times opposing muscles are supposed to fire to help control the movement, a phenomenon called co-contraction. Imagine that you are throwing a ball. Your triceps muscles in the back of your arm fire to straighten your arm for the throw. Unless your biceps, which are the opposite (reciprocal) muscles also fire (and not inhibit or relax), your arm cannot control how hard you throw, how fast you straighten your arm, or the precision of the throw. Reciprocal inhibition is not automatic or guaranteed to help your stretching. That means you don't need to tighten one side of a limb to loosen the other.

Do You Have to Hold All Stretches for 30 Seconds?

- It's not necessary to hold every stretch for a minimum of 30 seconds. In treatment for some injuries, holding a lengthened position is sometimes used to stop certain internal receptors from firing. For restoring healthy resting length and retraining healthy positioning using many of the stretches in this book, holding for at least a few seconds is enough. In this way you can easily get the benefit of doing dozens of stretches to restore healthy posture and movement ability in a few minutes, several times a day, without changing clothes, going to a gym, or stopping your day. Stretch often in a relaxed manner, training yourself to move easily, and then hold the healthy new length.

How Can I Remember How to Do All the Stretches Right?

- Many people labor to memorize lists of rules, positions, and joint angles for each stretch. Instead, know what you are trying to accomplish and see if you are moving in a way that does that. If you understand what the stretch is supposed to do, you can position yourself for the results. Do the purpose of the stretch, not a list of rules or steps to "do" a stretch.

Don't Undo Your Stretching With Bad Daily Habits

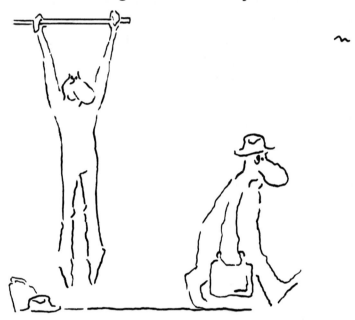

- After stretching to increase joint space and lengthen muscles, don't walk away slouching and compressing your joints. Doing a few stretches does not reverse the tightening and strain on your body from unhealthy movement during the rest of the day. When you walk away after your stretches, hold the healthy, increased joint space and good positioning.

Brain Stretch:

- When you use good positioning for daily life, you can stop the pain and injuries from chronic overstretching and from the tightening that occurs in the opposite areas.

Brain Stretch—What Does Stretching Do?

- Bears can hibernate without losing bone mass. Frogs can lie dormant under the ice without losing muscle. We can't stay healthy without movement. We need to move daily for joint, bone, circulatory, muscle and, even brain health. Astronauts in space lose bone and muscle from the lack of gravity making their muscles pull on their bones, no matter how much protein and calcium they eat. Limbs in a cast thin and weaken. Without movement, joints become damaged. Joints don't normally have a high blood supply. The way your joints receive food and oxygen and move wastes out is through movement. Prolonged bed rest (more than 2 days) weakens all the systems of the body. Over time, the weakening can become dangerous. It is important to be active.

- People often stretch to become flexible or healthy, but stretch in tight, strained, forced, unhealthy ways. Another problem is stretching in ways that do not stretch the area you think you are stretching. It is not a mystery when you don't become more flexible or prevent injuries. Use the healthy stretches and knowledge in this book to restore healthy resting and moving length to your muscles, so that you no longer stand and move with in strained, unhealthy positions. Use the stretches so that healthy standing and moving posture becomes comfortable.

- After gaining the flexibility and muscle length to stand and move in healthy positions, remember to stand and move in healthy positions. Stretching alone does not fix your posture. Intelligent stretching makes healthy positioning comfortable. Then you hold it. Plenty of flexible people have poor posture, pain, and injuries. It is also not the case that strengthening alone fixes joint pain or injuries. Many strong people have unhealthy posture, and the back, neck, and other pain and injuries that go with it. Use stretching to train healthy movement, then breathe, smile, relax, and move in healthy ways.

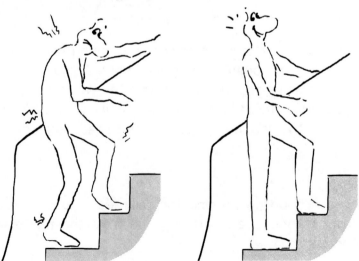

Use Daily Life as Your Stretching:

- When going up the stairs, keep your heel down on the upper step as you step up, for healthy Achilles and leg stretch with each step.

- When you stand, stand straight to keep healthy length in the front of your hip instead of bending forward, arching your lower back, or tipping your hip, which pressures your lower back and tightens your hip.

- Keep your shoulders from slouching or hunching forward, to get built-in stretch and exercise for your upper back. Don't force your shoulders back so much that you make your back and neck hurt.

- When you notice your shoulders tightening and hunching upward when cooking, working, exercising, driving, and other activities, breathe and tell yourself, "Relax shoulders down."

- When going down the stairs, keep your heel down longer on the upper step, rather than picking your heel up immediately. Keeping your weight back toward your heel is more stable, keeps the effort on your leg muscles and off your knee joints, and stretches the back of your legs. Step down lightly. Use leg muscles to decelerate, so that you get a gentle stretch with each step, instead of straining and jarring.

- For all the many times every day that you bend for things, bend your knees. When you bend for things with your feet side-by-side, bend your knees keeping your heels down on the floor for the entire bend, to stretch your calf muscle and Achilles tendon. When you bend with one foot in front of the other, keep your front heel on the floor and your front knee over your heel, not forward of your foot. Keep your back upright to avoid the loading and overstretching that adds to back pain.

- When you sit, sit up instead of letting your hip roll and curl under you. By sitting upright, you will get a stretch in the back of your hip and will reduce the pressure on your lower back discs.

- When getting in and out of chairs, keep your heels down, and try not to bow far forward. Sit down lightly, using leg muscles. Improve balance (safely) by not using your hands.

- When you sit on the floor, sit up straight. Make sure you can move your pelvis and hip straight so that you do not sit with your hip rolled under you. Try getting up without pushing off your hands. These are basic, not advanced, human movement skills.

- When you walk, keep both feet facing straight ahead, not turned inward or outward. Walking straight gives built-in real-life (functional) foot and Achilles tendon stretch with each step.

- Whenever you reach overhead, don't let your lower back increase the normal arch. Don't lean the upper body back. Preventing overarching prevents lower back pain from hyperlordotic (overarched) pressure. Reaching up without arching from your lower back gives a better stretch in your shoulder and functional core training from holding neutral spine.

Stretch Smarter Stretch Healthier

- Functional stretching isn't doing sets and reps of stretches, or holding for set lengths of time, then going back to unhealthful positioning in daily life.

- Think of healthful joint positioning and body mechanics like toilet training. You hold it, even when you don't feel like it. Use healthy positioning all the time for real life, and you won't get stiff and sore in the first place. Don't tighten yourself all day, then use stretching as something you stop your day and change clothes to do for a set time, then go back to a tight, strained life of bad positioning, and wondering why you hurt or are tight even though "you stretch."

- With the information in this book, you can understand what determines healthy positioning, then apply that knowledge to make all your stretches functional and your daily activities healthier.

- With the information in this book, you can stretch smarter, stretch healthier, and then use it for all you do.

Credits

- Front cover photos © 2006 Arttoday.com and Jupiter Images
- Back cover and author photos by Paul Plevakas
- Drawings by Jolie Bookspan Plevakas and Todd Sargood

Books and Resources by Dr. Jolie Bookspan

Fun classes, programs, Fitness Fixer health column, Academy of Functional Exercise Medicine (AFEM), and books: **www.DrBookspan.com**

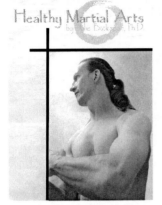

Healthy Martial Arts
Huge wealth of information for all athletes. Top level book for training body and mind. Winner of the EUSA International Martial Arts Black Belt Hall of Fame Readers Choice Award. 232 pages. Over 200 photos. Beautiful print edition and full color e-Book.

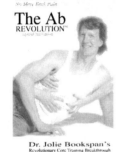

The Ab Revolution™ No More Crunches No More Back Pain. New Third edition expanded. Groundbreaking core training method used by military, athletes, and top spine docs. Step-by-step instructions, 114 drawings and photos. 131 pages. Print edition and color e-Book.

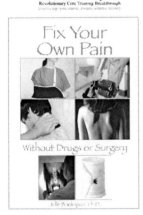

Fix Your Own Pain Without Drugs or Surgery
Back pain, neck pain, shoulder, knee, foot, ankle, wrist, and hip pain, problem toes, plantar fasciitis, disc pain, herniated disc, sciatica, lordosis, impingement, spondylolisthesis, flat feet, leg cramps, muscle pain. It's all here. Drawings and photos. 330 pages.

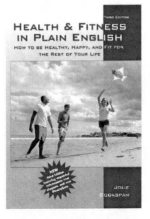

Health & Fitness in Plain English New THIRD revised edition - **How to be Healthy Happy and Fit for the Rest of Your Life.**
Replaces 1st and 2nd editions. All-in-one book, thirty-one fun chapters of fitness, nutrition, health, disease prevention, fixing back and neck pain, joint pain, functional exercise, "green" fitness, stretching, and fun facts about the body. 371 pages, illustrated.

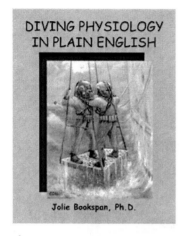

Diving Physiology in Plain English

The book for every scuba diver, novice to instructor. New blue cover edition replaces old green cover book. Fun understanding of decompression, computers, heat and cold, diving injuries, diving fitness, diving medicine, gender, fun facts, full glossary. 246 pages, illustrated.

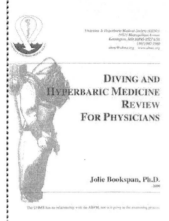

Diving and Hyperbaric Medicine Review For Physicians

Reviews the entire field in quick bulleted summaries. Includes sample American Board of Preventive Medicine (ABPM) board exam questions in each area to prepare for board certification, plus decompression calculations, and chamber protocols. Complete reference for anyone, physician or non. 226 pages.

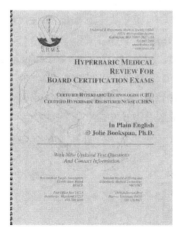

Hyperbaric Medical Review For Certified Hyperbaric Technologist (CHT) and Certified Hyperbaric Registered Nurse (CHRN)

Easy review for hyperbaric chamber nurses and technicians. Includes TCom module, and sample board exam questions and answers to study for the CHT and CHRN certification tests. Updated test questions with answers, step by step calculations, and explanations, all in Plain English. 190 pages.

PLUS

The Fitness Fixer. Free, electronic health column. Making exercise, medicine, and fitness healthy. Several new techniques weekly.

Academy of Functional Exercise Medicine (AFEM)—International Academy to make people, communities, and practice of medicine healthier. Certification, Fellow advancement, classes, projects, awards, fun.

About the Author

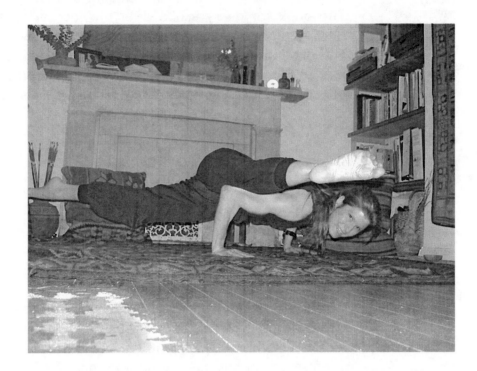

Dr. Bookspan is a former professor of anatomy and physiology, and military research scientist in extreme physiology, also called environmental physiology, which is the study of how the human body works during exposures to extremes — heat, cold, altitude, immersion, high G-forces, injury states, exercise, weightlessness, high pressure atmosphere, and forensics. Her life work is to develop methods for top training with reduced injuries. She put her techniques to work as an undefeated full contact martial artist and national-class swimmer, and to rehab from two (non-fighting) accidents that left her unable to walk for years—twice. Her techniques are used around the world by military teams, top athletes, and medical centers.

CPSIA information can be obtained at www.ICGtesting.com
Printed in the USA
LVOW09s1016190115

423323LV00004B/86/P

9 780972 121460